ADVANCE PRAISE FOR *CARING MATTERS MOST*

"Mark Lazenby is right: Caring matters most. Yet we find ourselves in a rapidly changing health care system that seems more chaotic, stressful and uncaring than ever before—and in a society that continues to devalue caring as the foundation of health and healing. This book holds the promise for ensuring that nurses are outspoken advocates for bringing the elements of caring into our health care organizations, systems, and policies. For both new and seasoned nurses who are concerned about the "business" of health care pushing out nurses' essential role and moral obligation to care for and about individuals, families and communities, *Caring Matters Most* is essential reading. It is also essential reading for anyone concerned about whether our health care system and those who work in it understand how to make caring our primary mission. If we don't, we are lost."

—Diana J. Mason, PhD, RN, FAAN, Senior Policy Service Professor,
George Washington University School of Nursing

"This 'little book' details the big ideas that form the foundation of the nursing profession. It is a must read for those new to the profession and those long in the profession alike. In simple but powerful prose Mark Lazenby reminds us why we nurse and what it means to be a nurse."

—Judith B. Krauss, MSN, RN, FAAN, Dean and Professor Emerita,
Yale University, School of Nursing

"A crucial book for all nurses, novice or experienced, it made my heart sing and brought tears to my eyes. Lazenby says to be a nurse is to be 'compelled to care' and he beautifully details the ethics of that compulsion. Read *Caring Matters Most* to remember why we do this challenging, but ever so important, job of nursing."

—Theresa Brown, PhD, BSN, RN, *New York Times* best-selling author of
The Shift: One Nurse, Twelve Hours, Four Patients' Lives

"Noble and often moving. An eloquent argument that caring, not reasoned principles, enables each of us to work towards a better world."

—Richard A. Burton, MD, Author of *On Being Certain:*
Believing You Are Right Even When You're Wrong

"Many have recommended the ethics of care as an approach to nursing ethics. Lazenby has provided an excellent account of what the ethics of care actually means for practitioners of the profession. His broadly Aristotelian approach begins by describing the ethical habits of a caring nurse. His approach is fresh and interesting; personal as well as erudite. He is a philosopher, but he writes as a nurse for his fellow nurses, providing dozens of concrete examples of caring in action. A perfect book for nursing ethics students or anyone interested in the ethics of care and the healing professions."

—Daniel Sulmasy, MD, PhD, MACP, Member, Presidential
Commission for the Study of Bioethical Problems

"Good nursing, Mark Lazenby reminds us, needs attentive care by trustworthy nurses, which regulatory requirements and formal accountability can never replace. A humane and timely reminder."

—Onora O'Neill, The Baroness O'Neill of Bengarve

"Mark Lazenby reconnects nurses to their moral core—caring for and about the welfare of others. He invites readers to transcend a narrow definition of ethics as application of principles to embodying our values in moment-to-moment presence and action."

—Cynda Hylton Rushton PhD, RN, FAAN, Anne and George L. Bunting
Professor of Clinical Ethics, Johns Hopkins University
Berman Institute of Bioethics & School of Nursing

CARING MATTERS MOST

The Ethical Significance of Nursing

By

Mark Lazenby, PhD, APRN, FAAN

ASSOCIATE PROFESSOR OF NURSING

YALE UNIVERSITY SCHOOL OF NURSING

NEW HAVEN, CT

OXFORD

UNIVERSITY PRESS

OXFORD
UNIVERSITY PRESS

Oxford University Press is a department of the University of Oxford. It furthers the University's objective of excellence in research, scholarship, and education by publishing worldwide. Oxford is a registered trade mark of Oxford University Press in the UK and certain other countries.

Published in the United States of America by Oxford University Press 198 Madison Avenue, New York, NY 10016, United States of America.

© Oxford University Press 2017

Library of Congress Cataloging-in-Publication Data
Names: Lazenby, Mark, author.
Title: Caring matters most : the ethical significance of nursing / by Mark Lazenby.
Description: New York, NY : Oxford University Press, [2017] |
Includes bibliographical references and index.
Identifiers: LCCN 2016031479 | ISBN 9780199364541 (pbk.)
Subjects: | MESH: Nurse-Patient Relations | Empathy | Ethics, Nursing |
Nurses—psychology
Classification: LCC RT86.3 | NLM WY 88 | DDC 610.7306/99—dc23
LC record available at https://lccn.loc.gov/2016031479

1 3 5 7 9 8 6 4 2

Printed by Webcom, Inc., Canada

For Donna's memory and for Ruth

DISCLAIMER

The clinical stories I have told in this book are faithful to my experiences and to what I have been told by other nurses, but I have changed the particularities of real events such that they would not be recognizable, except those stories that are about me and my family.

CONTENTS

CONTENTS

PART II
THE ETHICAL SIGNIFICANCE OF NURSES' LIVES

FOREWORD

Mark Lazenby has written a brilliant book on the ethical significance and moral sources of nursing. This book articulates everyday ethics and moral sources in nursing that are profoundly true to the practice and profession of nursing. While fresh and original, this work lies deeply in the best traditions of nursing practice and theory. I believe that most nurses will resonate to the truths demonstrated in the examples taken directly from the author's own and other nurses' practice. This work combines the ideals and reality of nursing in highly original ways, ways that do not look to "outsiders" for the strength and imagination that nurses themselves possess in their practice. Instead, the nurse-author looks within the powers and imagination of nurses themselves. Lazenby offers a critique and a way out of the unreasonable demands and injustices that patients and nurses encounter in hierarchical, impersonal health care systems. He notes that, through partnering with patients, nurses can make the health care system more just and humane. Lazenby states (in Chapter 10),

> In the United States, nursing is the largest profession among the
> health care professions, and among all the occupations in the

United States, it is second in the number of people employed in it. We are many, and we touch many, many more lives. To bring about the good society among the many lives we touch, we first must bring it about among ourselves. Our work to bring about the good society for all starts with bringing about the good society among the community of nurses, a community in which we treat all nurses with respect. Moreover, we continue to empower ourselves among other health care professions when we build a civil community for ourselves.

In the National Carnegie Study of Nursing Education we found that nurses explicitly described nursing ethics in terms of bioethics; specifically, students and faculty recited ethical principles such as justice, truth-telling, beneficence, and patient autonomy and rights. Yet in their first-person, experience-near narratives, nurses told of the centrality of understanding and being with the patient as a person, of preserving the patient's identity and personhood in the midst of depersonalized health care. This kind of gap between formal principles and actual practice is preferable to practice falling below principles. In the Carnegie study, we found that lived understandings and practices captured in first-person, experience-near narratives were more nuanced and better informed than explicit principles and beliefs that student nurses had learned in their classes on ethics. Mark Lazenby's book fills in this gap between the lived practice of nursing, the ethos, and the formal explicit principles and beliefs about good nursing practice typically taught in nursing ethics classes. He takes a strong stance that principles not instantiated in practice cannot capture the moral imagination and notions of good in the best nursing practice.

The first part of the book describes the following moral sources and habits of good nursing practice: trustworthiness, imagination, beauty, space, and presence are each described and illustrated as moral sources and the everyday ethos of nursing practice. Because nurses meet patients/clients in situations of potential vulnerability, first and foremost nurses must be trustworthy. Following the philosopher Onora O'Neill, Lazenby exemplifies how trustworthiness involves competence, reliability, and honesty between nurses and their patients/clients. Without clinical and moral imagination, nurses cannot bridge gaps between patient concerns and possibilities by taking concrete actions in response to what the patient would be and do if he or she had complete powers of intent and action. Here, Lazenby draws on the wisdom of Virginia Henderson:

> The unique function of the nurse is to assist the individual, sick or well, in the performance of those activities contributing to health or its recovery (or to a peaceful death) that he would perform unaided if he had the necessary strength, will or knowledge. And to do this in such a way as to help him gain independence as rapidly as possible.

What nurses now do through masterful management of physiological functions through medications and technology exceeds what was possible when Virginia Henderson wrote this account of the unique functioning of nursing, but the truth of the functions of nursing practice remains unchanged with the expansions of nursing interventions. The goal is still patient recovery, empowerment, and maximizing patient/client powers. The responsibilities and accountabilities of nurses are dramatically increased with the new technical and medical possibilities, but the goal remains the same: restoration of the patient's own powers to the extent possible.

I am inspired in reading the moral sources of beauty and goodness through drawing on beauty for strength, imagination, and positive growth for patients and nurses in the midst of illness and vulnerability. By seeing beauty in the aliveness of patients, their strengths and imagination for living in the midst of vulnerability, we find one of the most pervasive moral sources for imagination in nursing practice. As Lazenby writes in Chapter 1,

> I use Elaine Scarry's work on beauty and justice to argue that the habit of beauty—that is, the habit of seeing patients' aliveness as beautiful—is a habit that cultivates in us the moral character of nursing. When we think of an object as beautiful, we are compelled to promote its beauty, or when it has been injured, to restore it. The same is true of people. In her essay "The Nurse," Goodrich writes that nurses work in the interstices between science and philosophy, interstices in which facile answers to life's enduring questions and problems cannot be found.

Lazenby illustrates drawing on beauty for nursing imagination in actual caring practices of nurses, both his own and others. As a nurse, I resonate to the beauty described and experienced in the practice of nursing.

Both social–relational and physical spaces for healing are described as essential for the everyday caring practices of nurses. Social–relational spaces cannot be created without attentiveness and having the patient matter as a person with concerns, beauty, and vulnerabilities. In the social–relational spaces we create, nurses mitigate some of the impersonal and bureaucratic social spaces of today's health care institutions. In these social spaces of healing and vulnerability we are privileged to meet others as one of us in our common humanity.

Finally, Lazenby addresses the art of presence essential to all caring practices in nursing. He describes in Chapter 1 nurses' moral stance of being in the world in caring practices:

The habits of trustworthiness, imagination, beauty, space, and presence come together in individual nurses who, through living these habits, embody the profession's moral character.

Trustworthy nursing practice; a beautiful image of a sick person restored to health, a potentially sick person's health promoted, or a dying person's aliveness preserved until death; the creation of an inhabitable space for patients to be who they are, undefined by disease and disorder; and the presence of nurses in the lives of people who need care.

We find few authors willing to tackle the task of putting into words the moral sources and ideals of nursing practice through examples of the best nursing practice as well as examples of our best practices in the midst of imperfect worlds of practice. In the examples and stories, the ideal and real are not split in oppositional ways but rather integrated. Lazenby takes on the imperfect work environments and unreasonable demands encountered by nurses, from the stance of a nurse who has experienced these demands firsthand. In the midst of the unreasonable demands Lazenby calls on imagination. I am reminded that skydivers seldom complain about the terrors and dangers of their craft. Instead, they focus on the highs of flying above the Earth, the challenges, and the amazing vistas. Meeting others in our common humanity of vulnerabilities, enlivening beauty, and strength is a privilege. I am inspired to be a better nurse by reading this book.

I hope that *Caring Matters Most: The Ethical Significance of Nursing* will become the essential text for an ethic of caring taught in all nursing schools.

Patricia Benner, RN, PhD, FAAN

PREFACE

I recently sat with my son in a university's large lecture hall. It was full of high school seniors and their parents. We were there for an admissions information session. The admissions officer leading the session asked the crowd to name the college major that had the highest median starting salary upon graduation. People, mostly parents, started yelling out names of typically high-paying professions. But no one whom I could hear yelled out "nursing," though I said it loud enough for my son to take notice. The admissions officer corrected the crowd. "It is nursing," he said. He went on to say that the median starting salary for new graduates from that university's Bachelor of Science in Nursing program was a full twenty thousand dollars a year more than the median starting salary for new graduates from the university's other undergraduate programs. With surprise in their voices, many in the room replied with "Oh!" Some parents turned toward their children with a look that said, "Maybe you should apply to nursing!" I wanted to stand up and say—with pride—that I am a nurse and that we are highly educated health care professionals. We have university degrees. We have studied the sciences, the liberal arts, and the subject matter of our field. "You shouldn't be shocked that we make good salaries!" But I also wanted to caution any would-be nursing applicants: "Nursing is not just a well-paid job. It is a highly technical, demanding profession in which often, very often, you hold the balance of another person's life in your hands. And because what you do as a nurse matters so much, it is a profession with a moral character at the heart of its identity."

I wrote *Caring Matters Most* to explore this moral character. I did so through a nontraditional logic, a logic centered on ways of working and living as a nurse, not on decision-making algorithms. Using this "psychological logic," I tell stories—my own and those of others—that delve into the relationships nurses have with patients and families, with themselves, with each other, and with the world. For it is in telling and listening to each other's stories in everyday plain language (the language I try to use) that we learn about each other's moral conflicts and how to respond to these conflicts with the moral character of the profession.

Nursing has a unique moral character. It is a character centered on caring for others and for the world. This character is the reason I became a nurse. As a nurse, I have come to believe that nursing demands more of me than merely caring for others. It demands that I think about my own moral life. For being a good nurse involves the commitment to being a good person, a person whose daily life centers on caring.

This is what I wanted to say to the high school seniors sitting in that university lecture hall: "Go ahead! Declare nursing as your major. But be forewarned. If you become a nurse, you will take on an identity in which caring becomes your way of life. If you become a nurse, being a good person will necessarily involve caring for patients and families, for yourself, for other nurses, and for the world."

If you are considering becoming a nurse, I hope you come away from reading this book with a sense of the joy and deep satisfaction that a life of caring brings. If you are nursing student, I hope you come away with the realization that, to be a good nurse, technical skill is necessary but insufficient: to be a good nurse, you must be a good person. If you are a nurse, I hope you find in this book confirmation of the good life of nursing. If you are not a nurse and do not intend to become one, I hope you come to see nurses as good people who, through their daily acts of caring, make the world a better place.

Mark Lazenby
August 25, 2016

ACKNOWLEDGMENTS

My first word of thanks goes to Gwynedd-Mercy College for inviting me in spring of 2013 to give a set of lectures on nursing and the good society. These lectures started a current of thought and effort that I then pursued in lectures I gave at Yale School of Nursing in the winter terms of 2015 and 2016 to Doctor of Nursing Practice students. What sets Yale nursing students apart is not so much their intelligence, though they are exceedingly smart, but their dedication to making the world a better place. They have improved my thinking about how nursing can bring about good in the world; I thank them.

As ever, I thank my Yale colleagues with whom I have discussed these matters. Tish Knobf, my division chair, has been gracious with her encouragement and support. Marjorie Funk has always had a sympathetic ear, the sign of a true friend. Donna Diers told me, in no uncertain terms, that I had to write this book. She died before I could even begin. Her charge kept me going. Ruth McCorkle has been my teacher, mentor, and friend; I have talked through many of these ideas with her in conversations that improved my thinking, and from her, I have learned what it means to be a great and a good nurse.

Andrea Knobloch and Rebecca Suzan, my editors at Oxford University Press, deserve my thanks for their forbearance and support. Leonie Gombrich, book nurse-midwife extraordinaire, has brought to bear her sharp mind, editorial skills, good humor, and inimitable patient persistence to the writing of this book, making sure that my thoughts do not arouse the guffaws of critics and my English prose the consternation of readers. Though this is a little book, it was a most difficult book to write. It required longer incubation of thought than I anticipated and complete honesty of heart and mind. Leonie, I could not have completed it without you; you gave me the gumption—and at times the strongest of nudges—to pull from the deepest wells within; thank you. Any superficialities, lacunae, errors of thought, or infelicitous prose that remain are my fault alone. Finally, and certainly not least, my wife and son have been my wholly tolerable supporters—and encouragers—of my philosophy of nursing endeavors; to Jodi and Ethan especially, my thanks and my love.

EPIGRAPH

The unique function of the nurse is to assist the individual, sick or well, in the performance of those activities contributing to health or its recovery (or to a peaceful death) that he would perform unaided if he had the necessary strength, will or knowledge. And to do this in such a way as to help him gain independence as rapidly as possible.

—Virginia Henderson

PART I

THE ETHICAL SIGNIFICANCE OF NURSING

Chapter 1

The Moral Character of Nursing

When I was considering becoming a nurse, I was a grown man with a family of my own and, with a book just published, a good career in philosophy ahead of me. But in the aftermath of both my parents' early deaths, deaths that followed protracted periods of illness, my mind kept going back to my final year of secondary school. That year, I had taken a yearlong night course on basic nursing at the hospital of the small town in which I lived. It truly was a small-town hospital, with fewer than fifty beds, no intensive care unit, and an emergency room that served as a way station for people who needed to be transported to a major medical center, the closest of which was more than a two-hour drive away. But there, I first witnessed nurses' commitment to caring for patients, their families, and their community. There, among those small-town hospital nurses, I witnessed the moral character of nursing. Those nurses cared.

Aristotle, in both the *Eudemian Ethics* and the *Nichomachean Ethics*, uses the word "ethics" to refer to moral character. The Greek word he uses for it is ἔθος, which, when translated, is *ethos*. To put it in modern terms, moral character is one's ethos. Those nurses who taught me basic nursing in my last year of secondary school all shared the same ethos. It was nursing's ethos, the ethos of caring.

The nurses of my hometown hospital cared about each patient's life, and they cared with joy. I thought of them as a group of Mother Teresas. Of course, I was young and did not see their grumpy moments or hear their dissatisfactions. But as I was processing the years of my parents' chronic illnesses and untimely deaths, I asked myself what I wanted to do with the rest of my life, and I remembered the moments I had witnessed the moral character of nursing among those small-town hospital nurses. They practiced nursing as though it were a vocation. I began questioning whether I wanted to move on from philosophy to become a nurse. Was it a vocation to which I felt called?

A vocation, the American essayist and novelist Frederick Buechner writes, "is the kind of work (*a*) that you need most to do and (*b*) that the world needs most to have done." Buechner's definition guided my questioning. Doing the kind of work that you need most to do means that it is what you must do if you are to be joyful in life. It is the kind of work that gives you a sense of completeness. Would nursing bring me the joy I had seen among those small-town hospital nurses as they did their work, the joy of doing work without which my life would be incomplete?

It seemed to me that the work of nursing would indeed bring me joy, and I wanted that joy; but I felt the weight of what nursing would require of me. If I were to become a nurse, it would be more than a job that pays a good wage, more even than a challenging career that would allow for advancement or, even, intellectual stimulation, though nursing as a profession does all this. As a nurse, I would be compelled to care.

When you are compelled to care—that is, when nursing is something without which your life would be incomplete—nursing becomes a principle within you. It becomes something you *must* do; you have no other choice. You cannot turn away from, or fail to see, those who need care. You cannot forbid them to come into your life. Rather, the moral character of nursing becomes an internal principle that guides your every action. Nursing becomes who you are—not just in your outside profession but deep inside, in your character. Nursing's character becomes yours. Your actions become governed by an internal principle you hear in your heart and mind when you say, "I am a nurse." When nursing becomes your vocation, caring becomes most important.

Annie Warburton Goodrich is one of the founders of university-based nursing education. In her conception of nursing, she characterizes the profession as being concerned with creating "a better world." For Goodrich, working during the progressive era of the 1920s and 1930s, this better world is a world not riven by war, a world in which the integrating force of common humanity overcomes the borders of countries. It is a world of equality, especially for women and children. Hospitals are accessible to all, and the care is so scientifically based and precisely delivered that no patient has to stay longer than is absolutely necessary. Nursing care brings about this better world by lessening the vulnerabilities that lead to inequalities and threaten life. Nurses care for the sick until they are well and the dying, to give them the best life possible for as long as possible. Goodrich's view of nursing is one in which nurses care about creating a better world.

But the moral character of nursing encompasses more than the feeling of caring. It involves caring in such a way that the better world is realized. The action of caring brings about a better world.

Caring is not unique to nursing. Physicians care. So do pharmacists and physical and occupational therapists and nutritionists and massage therapists and social workers and psychologists. Indeed, health care professionals of all stripes care. If caring is not limited to nursing, as surely it is not, then what is the kind of caring that gives nursing its moral character?

Other health care professionals can faithfully fulfill the duties of their work without intimately caring for patients and communities. They most certainly may, but caring is not the essence of their work. Managing complex medical situations, performing surgery with exquisite precision, accurately dispensing medications, performing the appropriate therapeutic intervention—these are the duties of other health care professionals. But for us nurses, the heart of our profession is caring. We cannot not care and still be a good nurse.

When I thought of becoming a nurse and I looked back upon my experiences with the nurses in my hometown, I realized that they were not just kind and compassionate nurses, though they were certainly that. They were also good nurses, nurses who answered to the internal principle of their calling. Becoming a nurse would mean that I too would *have* to be a nurse in the same way. My acts of nursing care would have to be performed in such a way that they would be kind and compassionate, yes, but also moral: good acts. That is just what the vocation of nursing is: a vocation with a profound morality built into its very nature. In a real sense, nursing would be work that I had to do—work that I was morally bound to do.

Caring about and for others is a specific kind of calling. As the philosopher-nurse Patricia Benner says, the calling of nursing demands that we care "for the disenfranchised, the vulnerable, and the suffering." Given for whom we care, we build relationships that "protect [people] in their vulnerability while fostering growth and limiting vulnerability." People who are disenfranchised, vulnerable, sick, and dying, because of the circumstances they find themselves in, require more from us than they do from other relationships. They require that we care *about* and *for* them in ways that protect them, improve their lives, and convey that they matter.

What does it mean that you must care about and for others? It can mean giving your very life. Nurses in West Africa during the

Ebola crisis of 2014 cared about and for the sick stricken by the Ebola virus in this morally bound way. So overwhelmed by the magnitude of the outbreak, the inadequacies of the health care system, and the deaths of so many of her nurses, a head nurse on an infectious disease ward in Sierra Leone confessed that she had thought of quitting rather than continuing to care for people with Ebola. On top of it all, revolting nurses, overcome by Ebola's decimation of their colleagues, threatened her life, saying that she should prepare to die if another nurse on the ward died from Ebola. But she had no option, she said; she had to "go and save others." Nursing is a "calling," she said: she had to care about and for the sick in order to be true to herself. If she stopped caring, she would not be true to her internal principle, for surely she believed deep down that nursing is part of the work the world needs most to have done. If she did not care about and for Ebola patients, even in the face of the prospect of her own death at the hands of disgruntled nurses or through the virulence of Ebola itself, she would not be a *good* nurse.

All human beings carry the potential for vulnerability, not just Ebola patients and not just nurses caring for Ebola patients. People in high places, when life-limiting disease comes upon them, become vulnerable. Children, because of their incomplete physical, emotional, and intellectual maturity, are vulnerable. Patients, by virtue of being within byzantine health care systems that favor people who do not need health care, are vulnerable. The poor, the politically and socially disenfranchised, those afflicted by war, the physically or mentally disabled, the sick, the potentially sick lost in the system, by virtue of their vulnerability, lay claim to a special relationship, a relationship of caring about and for them in their vulnerability, until such time as they no longer need our care.

However, when we think of ethics and nursing, we do not always think of lessening vulnerability. It is tempting, rather, to think of ethics as a part of our nursing care only when dealing with situations in which not all people involved agree upon the way to proceed. When we think of ethics in this way, we apply the principles of bioethics in order to navigate the treacherous waters of such situations, which some refer to as ethical dilemmas. The four principles of bioethics, which the philosophers Tom Beauchamp and James Childress first articulated in *The Principles of Bioethics* in 1977, are autonomy, non-maleficence (do no harm), maleficence (do good), and justice. However, even when the parties involved in so-called ethical dilemmas apply the principles of bioethics, disagreement about the "right" way to proceed can persist. Indeed, what defines a dilemma is that reasonable people disagree on the "right" course of action. This is because the notion of "right" is relative to what a person holds as having absolute value. Take one of the most difficult dilemmas in clinical care, the dilemma in which a family does not want to disconnect a loved one from life support and the health care team wants to because it does not think the patient will ever recover. In these situations, the family and the health care team operate with different beliefs about what is of absolute value. Because of this, they have different interpretations of the "right" course of action. One resolution to this dilemma is for the health care team to have three "experts" agree on the course of action to take and overrule the family. When this happens, the clinicians who overrule the family are assured of their "right" application of the principles of bioethics, although the family continues to disagree. In dilemmas in which the principles of bioethics are supposed to provide us with clarity of action, the principles can lead us to believe that we have found the "right" way. Yet the "right" way is not absolute; if it were, the situation would not pose a dilemma in the first place, for all would agree upon the way to proceed. The problem with the principles of bioethics is that they dupe us into believing we are right in our course of action in an absolute way, not in a relative way. That is, they lead us to perform on ourselves the sleight of hand of believing that that which is relative is absolute.

If the principles of bioethics are of no real help in ethics, then how ought we proceed?

Beauchamp and Childress themselves suggest a way forward. They say that "what counts most in the moral life is not consistent adherence to principles . . . but reliable character." Ethical application of principles, after all, first requires ethical people. That is, moral character guides action, not only in situations in which a straightforward way to proceed is unclear but in everyday clinical care.

Most of us come to nursing with our own beliefs about how we ought to act. We came to these beliefs through our families of origin, through our religion or culture, through reading and learning about how good people lived, through mentors who influenced us along life's way, or through our own moral compass, whose bearings we have figured out in the school of life. The Greek word Aristotle uses for "habit" (ἠθική), when transliterated from the Greek, is *ethike*. It is the adjectival form of "ethos" (ἔθος), the word for moral character. A habit is an outward behavior that shows forth an inward devotion. We sometimes call these behaviors habits of the heart or habits of mind, the kind of habits that show others our truest selves. When speaking about ethics, habits show forth our moral character. This is true for us not just in our personal lives but in our professional lives as nurses. The habits of a good nurse show forth the profession's moral character of caring about and for people.

Something very profound happens when we look at ethics and nursing this way. That which *is* good about nursing (nursing's moral character) and the *ought* of nursing (the habits by which we ought to practice) become one. This cohering of the "ought" and the "is" of nursing is the profession's deepest core, its truest expression, that what we are and what we do are the same thing. This distinguishes the profession of nursing from other health care professions. Caring is the ultimate point of reference for what we do as nurses. It is that which gives our acts of nursing ethical significance. This fundamental moral commitment to caring is where the actions of an individual nurse are grounded in the moral character of the profession. In this way, ethics is not a separate academic or professional discipline reserved for those specially trained in bioethics, but rather, ethics is inherent in nursing. It is not ethics *and* nursing; it is the ethics *of* nursing.

Ethical dilemmas do arise in health care. New technologies do pose concerns, for example, in research on humans, human tissue, and animals. We do need experts in bioethics to help us think about these concerns. However, ethics cannot be split off from everyday nursing. When we talk about ethics in the context of everyday nursing, we talk about the good of what we do—the good of caring about and for the sick, the potentially sick, and the dying. It is not that the profession of nursing is without any other commitments. It is, rather, that without caring about people in their vulnerabilities, and caring for them with the aim of bringing about for them in the here and now a better world—without the fundamental commitment to caring as the greatest thing—nursing is not nursing. Others in the health care professions can do their jobs without both caring about and for patients and their communities, but nurses cannot. Good nurses embody this moral character, and from them we learn that caring is primary, as I learned from those nurses in my hometown hospital and from the story of that head nurse on the Ebola ward in West Africa.

Thinking about the ethics of nursing delves into the heart of nursing's moral character—into its ethos of caring. I do so in this book by investigating five habits that, when lived, embody the profession's ethos of caring. Although we may be able to think of other habits or characterize them in different ways, I suggest these five are sufficient to embody nursing's moral character.

In Chapter 2, I speak about the habit of trustworthiness. Drawing upon the work of the contemporary philosopher Onora O'Neill, I argue that trustworthiness is competent, reliable, and honest nursing care and care that is committed to fairness, that is, to equal access to the conditions of health. When we practice with competence, reliability, honesty, and fairness over and over, we develop in ourselves the habit of being trustworthy, a habit patients and communities take close notice of. This is, I suggest, why people rate nurses as among the most trusted of all the professions. Through our trustworthy professional touch, people recognize that, for us nurses, caring comes first.

Those nurses in my local hospital were trustworthy. We all knew it. Growing up, whenever one of us kids scraped our knee or bonked our head, our mother would dispatch one of us to go fetch the nurse who lived around the corner. Yet good nursing care requires more than trustworthiness. It also requires imagination.

In order to know what acts of nursing care to perform, we must imagine what patients would do for themselves to restore or promote their health, or to have a serene death. We have to care about them in such a way as to imagine better lives for them. This imagination—what some call moral imagination—directs care. Imagination is the second habit of the good nurse, which I explore in Chapter 3.

In my final year of secondary school, I saw the nurses use moral imagination before I knew what it was. Even more impressive, however, was the way they treated patients as if they were fully alive, no matter how sick they were or even if they were dying; they were alive, and the nurses cared that their patients were alive. That is, they saw the beauty of each patient.

In Chapter 4, I use Elaine Scarry's work on beauty and justice to argue that the habit of beauty—that is, the habit of seeing patients' aliveness as beautiful—is a habit that cultivates in us the moral character of nursing. When we think of an object as beautiful, we are compelled to promote its beauty, or when it has been injured, to restore it. The same is true of people. In her essay "The Nurse," Goodrich writes that nurses work in the interstices between science and philosophy, interstices in which facile answers to life's enduring questions and problems cannot be found. Through our work in this unsettling and vague area of life, we as nurses are "capable of increasing beauty" by bringing "greater perfection to humanity." The habit of seeing others—indeed, of seeing the aliveness of others—as beautiful motivates us to perform the work of nursing.

Patients and families come to us for nursing care. They come to us in their vulnerabilities and ask us to care about them and for them in order to achieve better health and better quality of life as they are sick and dying. But their vulnerabilities do not define them. Our caring about and for our patients opens up a space for them to be people not defined by their vulnerabilities. This opening up of a space for our patients to be people is the fourth habit that, I argue in Chapter 5, embodies in us nursing's moral character.

In Chapter 6, I discuss the habit of presence—the habit of being in the presence of another person. When we are in the presence of another person, we respect that person's capacity to make decisions and to be in relationships. Profoundly, as nurses, we respect that person's capacity to be in relationship with us. Being in the presence of another person is, in that moment, to care most about—and for—that person.

The habits of trustworthiness, imagination, beauty, space, and presence come together in individual nurses who, through living these habits, embody the profession's moral character. Trustworthy nursing practice; a beautiful image of a sick person restored to health, a potentially sick person's health promoted, or a dying person's aliveness preserved until death; the creation of an inhabitable space for patients to be who they are, undefined by disease and disorder; and the presence of nurses in the lives of people who need care—when we cultivate in ourselves these habits, we practice nursing as if caring is the greatest thing.

Bioethicists cannot teach nurses how to live the moral character of the profession of nursing. Nurses must do this in the everyday practices of nursing care by cultivating with and for each other the habits of a good nurse.

When I watched nurses care about and for my dying parents, I knew I had seen that kind of deep caring before. It was a unique kind of caring, not the caring of other health care professionals, not the caring of friends and family, though they all cared. I thought of where I had seen this kind of caring before: in my last year of secondary school among the nurses in that small-town hospital. I remembered, and when I remembered, I knew that I wanted to become a nurse. You know the end of the story. I became a nurse. But in the years of becoming one, I realized that the nurses who first taught me nursing were not just showing me what it means to be a good nurse, although we do learn to be good nurses from adopting the habits of good nurses. They were teaching me that caring matters most. This is the ethical significance of nursing.

Chapter 2

Trustworthiness

A young woman and her partner had their first baby two weeks ago. They're back in the hospital now. She just had a postpartum hemorrhage. She and her partner had wanted an all-natural childbirth—no drugs, no epidural, no oxytocin to stimulate her labor, and attended by a midwife. And she wanted to breastfeed as soon as her baby was born. She had dreamed of breastfeeding for as long as possible—until the child was 2 or 3 years old, she thought. But the birth proved difficult. The midwife had five other women laboring that night. She popped her head into the couple's room only a handful of times in the course of labor. A nurse was with the couple, but she had another woman laboring, too. And the couple had no prior relationship with the nurse. The couple, in the patient satisfaction survey that they filled out a few weeks after the hemorrhage, said they felt alone during labor. Twenty hours after labor began, the nurse sent in an anesthesiologist. He started an epidural. They hooked up the laboring woman to oxytocin and inserted a fetal monitor. The couple were told this *had* to be done. Ten hours later, the woman found herself in the operating room undergoing a cesarean section. She delivered a healthy boy, 9 pounds 14 ounces.

Two weeks later, however, the young mother found herself in the same operating room undergoing a dilatation and curettage to remove the retained placenta that had caused the hemorrhage. After the surgery, she and her partner heard that she had lost a lot of blood—a transfusion was necessary—but that the surgical team was able to stop the bleeding without removing her uterus. As soon as the new mother recovered from the anesthesia, she wanted to pump her breasts to get rid of the milk contaminated with drugs. It was night, and just after the two-hour surgery and long recovery, she was too weak to do it herself. There was no space in the hospital room for her partner and newborn son to stay over; they had to go home, and the father had to give his newborn son bottles of formula, which felt wrong to him. He knew his partner's dream was to breastfeed. He worried that this would confuse his son. Would his baby boy ever go back to suckling at the breast? The young mother told her night nurse that she had to pump the "bad milk" out of her breasts. "I have to get this out," she said. "I want to feed my baby naturally."

The nurse had three other patients that night. She knew it would be difficult to help this woman pump. It would be difficult, even, to get the pump and supplies into the woman's room, much less do it for her. But the nurse saw the new mother's sadness in her slumped shoulders. The nurse felt the new mother's loneliness; her baby, which by the natural order of things should have been at her bosom, was not even in the hospital. And the nurse sensed the new mother's urgency: if she stopped pumping, she could stop lactating; and besides, this drug-laced breast milk had to be purged.

Amid her busyness, the nurse was in the young mother's room every two hours. She sat by the bed and held the breast pump collection cups up to the young mother's breast for the twenty minutes it took to drain them. The nurse, a mother five times over, regaled the young mother with stories of her children: the poopy messes when they were young, the constantly sticky kitchen floor, the chaos of unfolded laundry, school lunches left on the counter after the bus had come. They laughed together so loudly that it drowned out the nurse's grumbling stomach. She hadn't had time for a meal break her entire shift.

A few weeks after the young woman made it home to her partner and newborn son, she sent a note to the hospital along with the patient satisfaction survey. She said that she had never trusted anyone as much as she trusted that nurse that night.

What does it mean to trust? Why did this young woman say she trusted that night nurse?

Gallup polls the American public every year on its perception of the trustworthiness of different professions. Nurses were first included in the survey in 1999, and since then, they have topped the list except for 2001, when they came second to firefighters, which Gallup attributes to the events of 9/11. Often referred to as the "most trusted professions survey," the survey asks respondents "to rate the honesty and ethical standards of people" in different fields. In this chapter, I want to consider why the public thinks nursing is the most trusted of the professions.

Certainly, this trust has to do with honesty, about which the survey explicitly asks. However, the trust the public puts in nurses (and firefighters, for that matter) is different from the trust it puts, or does not put, in other professions. There are professions we may not believe are honest—for example, politicians and lobbyists, who round out the bottom of the list. Although politicians and lobbyists may be well intentioned, we suspect they probably will say things just to win elections or to get the laws passed that they want. Also, we may not always believe that police (an honorable profession, to be sure) will keep us safe—for example, if we are people of color living in a racially riven neighborhood. Our lack of trust in certain professions may be because we do not believe that they will be honest or fair. However, when the public says it believes nursing is the most honest and ethical of the professions, I believe it is saying something broader than just that nurses are honest.

The relationship between patients and nurses is built upon patients' entrusting us with their whole selves—their physical bodies, their thoughts and emotions, and their deepest hopes and fears, in the most intimate of ways, such as holding breast pump cups up to a young, new mother's swollen breasts to pump out breast milk laced with anesthetics. It seems a simple act, but it is an act in which the mother entrusts the nurse with restoring the hope that she will feed her newborn son naturally. This relationship—this trusting relationship—depends on nurses being trustworthy and on patients making claims (demands, even) on nurses that require them to respond with trust.

Elemental to the trust the public places in nurses is that, over time, the profession has proven itself to be trustworthy. The philosopher Onora O'Neill says that trustworthiness involves competence, reliability, and honesty. Let us consider each of these elements in turn.

The profession has an accountability system that ensures that any nurse who passes the nursing board has the training, skills, and knowledge to perform the basic duties of nursing. This accountability system helps to ensure nurses' competence. The profession accredits nursing education programs at regular intervals. It sets national boards of nursing that nurses must pass, thus proving that they have the minimum knowledge necessary to perform the duties of a nurse. Because of this accountability system, the public has, over time, come to trust the competence of nurses. That is, the public has come to believe that those who are called nurses by the profession have the training, knowledge, and skills necessary to perform the duties of nursing care. However, the competence of nurses is ensured by more than the accountability system of accrediting agencies and national examinations. Nurses ensure each other's competence.

Nursing, as many of the health care professions, is learned at the elbow of expert nurses. These expert nurses teach novice nurses how to practice in complex clinical situations. The expert nurse will supervise the novice until the novice demonstrates her or his competence. The philosopher-nurse Patricia Benner has called this a progression from novice to expert, which she explains in five stages.

In the first stage, the novice nurse, just beginning and thus without much clinical experience to accompany her or his training, lacks confidence to make clinical judgments. She or he requires continual cues from an expert nurse mentor about what to do. After experience in actual clinical situations, she or he progresses to being an advanced beginner, the second stage. She or he has become more efficient and skillful in the areas of clinical practice in which she or he has had experience, and in these areas she or he needs fewer cues about what to do. After a while, the nurse becomes more efficient, coordinated, and confident; she or he is now in the third stage, which Benner calls the competent stage. In the next stage, the proficient stage, the nurse analyzes potential problems and plans ahead to address them. When the nurse has reached the fifth stage, the expert stage, she or he has an intuitive grasp of a situation and homes in on an aspect of the problem that is the most critical.

Mentoring makes Benner's novice-to-expert model work. The expert nurse mentors the novice nurse through the early stages. The community of expert nurses mentors competent and proficient nurses—and each other. As the nature of nursing care changes along with the constant development of science and technology, nurses must mentor each other to maintain competence. In fact, expert nurses go back to being novices in new and different areas of nursing practice—for example, new machines to use, new quality care standards to implement, new medications to administer. In these foreign territories of technical care, through training and mentoring, the once-expert but now-novice nurse progresses again through the stages to become expert.

The profession seeks to ensure the competence of nurses by accrediting nursing schools and colleges and by administering board examinations. Increasingly, over the last hundred years, formal qualification and mentoring structures have been and are being put in place to replace the informal workplace mentoring that still exists. But even when it is not formalized, the community of nurses in a workplace knows not to let a novice nurse practice solo. It would not be safe: he or she could cause harm to patients, which would, in turn, harm him or her and the profession. This system of mentoring nurses through the stages of competence is a part of the backbone of the profession's trustworthiness. The community of nurses takes ownership of the trustworthiness of the profession.

Thus, the accrediting bodies, the state boards or councils of nurses, and the community of nurses that make up the profession all seek to ensure the competence of those whom the profession calls a nurse. This competence-ensuring system, although formal in some respects and informal in others, works. The public has come to believe that nurses can do what they say they can do. Indeed, people rely upon nurses to be and do who they say they are and what they say they can do.

The public entrusts itself to be cared for by nurses because the profession of nursing has, time and time again, proven itself competent. The Gallup survey asks the public to rate "people in these different fields." I can imagine that when members of the public answer the survey question, they think of a specific instance in which they have met or had dealings with a person in that particular profession.

"What was it like for me when I was cared for by a nurse?" they might ask themselves, and it is this recollection on which their survey response depends. The public cannot always judge the competence of individual nurses. How can it know whether a specific nursing act was the right thing to do in a specific clinical situation? Sometimes expert nurses alone can answer the question of the competence of nurses. Thus, when not answering surveys but in the course of their lives, the public has to rely upon the profession's judgment that a nurse is competent. However, based on the accumulation of specific experiences the public has had with nurses, it believes it can rely upon the profession to ensure nurses' competence.

Reliability involves such proof. Nurses must show, over and over and over again, that they are competent. Yet reliability is more than repeated demonstration of competence. The reliability of others matters most when we are in a state of dependence—when we are vulnerable.

People need nurses when they are in a dependent state. They rely upon nurses to do what needs to be done to lessen that dependence. This kind of reliance involves entrusting nurses with that which is precious. They entrust us with their sick bodies—and their hopes that our acts of nursing care will restore health. They entrust us with their well bodies—and their hopes that we will help them to do what needs to be done to keep them well. They entrust us with their dying bodies—and their hopes that we will provide them safe passage from this life. They rely upon us to restore and to promote health or to lead them to a peaceful death.

The young, new mother relied upon her night nurse to restore in her the hope that she would breastfeed her newborn son again—after the hemorrhage. The mother placed her trust in the night nurse, and this trust involved relying upon the night nurse to do for the mother what the mother could not do for herself. And the night nurse followed through. She proved herself reliable. She came every two hours to perform the simple but profound act of holding the breast pump cups to pump out the drug-laced breast milk. She came every two hours to care for the precious gift of hope the mother entrusted her with. We do not entrust people with that which we deem most precious unless we believe we can rely upon them.

But here is where the notion of reliance gets tricky for nurses. Patients have no choice but to entrust us with their bodies and their hopes. The young, new mother had to rely upon her night nurse to help her restore her body to a nonmedicated state—and her hope of breastfeeding her newborn son. The night nurse could have responded any number of ways: the night nurse could not have helped the mother pump at all, claiming busyness with patients who had more physically critical needs; the night nurse could have helped her once or twice during the shift; or the night nurse could have helped the mother every two hours, as she did. Regardless of the response, the mother still entrusted the night nurse with the hope of returning to a healthy state. The mother did this before she even knew what the night nurse's response would be. It was a plea, as if to say, "I have this precious gift to entrust you with. Can I rely on you?" With this plea, patients call us to be reliable, and this has the effect of making us reliable. The best analogy I have is that, when I was young and in primary school, my mother would entrust me with the money I needed to buy my school lunch and to return the change to her after school. Once she gave me the money in the morning before I left the house for school, I could have chosen what I did with it. I could have stopped by the corner market on the walk to school to buy candy (as I may have done once or twice). But my mother's act of entrusting me day after day, and her disappointment when I did not prove reliable, built reliability within me. In the same way, patients, by entrusting us time and time again with that which is most precious to them, put us in the position in which we must decide to act reliably. Each time we respond reliably, we build within us the quality of being reliable. And each time, we confirm our patients'—and the public's—belief that we are reliable.

The public has come to trust the competence of nurses, and the profession ensures that this trust is not misplaced. The public also trusts that nurses are reliable. As I have argued, our patients call us to be reliable, reliable with their most precious gifts of health and hope. They trust that nurses will reliably change the dirty bed, protect patients from falling, advocate for patients when they need a change in care plan, and, upon peril of their own lives, care for patients with Ebola. What it means to be a good nurse, in response to this gift of trust, is *reliably* to perform competent acts of nursing care.

According to O'Neill, honesty rounds out the trio of qualities necessary for trustworthiness. Honesty, in O'Neill's thinking, is as much about the absence of deception as it is about truthfulness. Both are at work in the trustworthiness of nurses. At this most basic level, patients trust that we are truthful about what the clear liquid is in the syringe we hold and are about to put into their bodies. Patients also trust that we are truthful that the medication in the syringe is the medication that they are supposed to get. They have very little way of verifying these things. But they trust that we are truthful—that is, that we do not deceive our patients. Of course, there have been incidents in which nurses intentionally deceive patients about medication; these are criminal acts. And, of course, nurses do sometimes give the wrong medication at the wrong time and in the wrong dose. These errors are not errors of deception. Still, they endanger the precious gift of health patients entrust us with. The ethical wrong of these unintentional medical errors is that they do harm to what patients have entrusted us with and to the trusting relationship between nurses and patients.

Beyond O'Neill's definition of honesty, I propose a high-order notion of honesty, not predicated on the absence of deception or on adherence to the technical, medical aspects of nursing care. This broader understanding of honesty includes practicing in accordance with the belief that all people ought to have equal access to the conditions necessary for good health. That is, this broader understanding of honesty includes fairness.

The profession exhibits this fairness in three ways. First, nurses have little at stake financially in the business of health care; and thus, their motivation has less to do with financial gain than with providing competent and reliable care. Second, all patients are the same to nurses, regardless of wealth or social status. Patients simply are vulnerable people in need of care. Thus, nurses are free to *be for* that which provides health care for *all* people. Third, and for me most profound, the fairness of the profession is a concern for the poor and dispossessed—those whose conditions in life put them at risk of poorer health than those who have access to plentiful and healthful food, clean water, livable communities, and affordable quality health care. Nurses are fair in that they are for equal access to the conditions necessary for health—and for equal access to the health care that can make death peaceful. It is this kind of honesty that, I suggest, the public recognizes when it rates nursing as among the most trusted of the professions.

Competent, reliable, and honest (and fair) acts of nursing care carry with them ethical significance. We mentor each other into being experts at nursing care—and this is *good* for both nurses and patients. Patients call upon us to provide reliable nursing care—and this is *good* for both nurses and patients. And when we provide care, we provide the same care to everyone who needs it; we are fair—and this is *good* for both nurses and patients and for a just and equal society. The habit of performing trustworthy acts of nursing care is essential for generating the public's trust.

We now see how being in the habit of performing trustworthy acts of nursing care has an ethical significance: it adds to the storehouse of trust. Trust is necessary. Life, with all its uncertainties, is impossible without trust. "None of us knows what might happen even the next minute," the philosopher and novelist Paolo Coelho said, "yet we still go forward. Because we trust." Trust, seen as a necessity of life, thus becomes a component of good health—and a peaceful death. The more trust we as nurses engender in our everyday, trustworthy acts of nursing practice, the more we restore and promote health—and contribute to peaceful deaths. We create more trust, and in a time and age in which suspicion and fear of harm are great, creating more trust is *good*.

This is what we do in our everyday, trustworthy acts of nursing practice, and it is our ethical duty. That is, we have a duty to engender trust and to use the trust we have engendered for the good of society. To fulfill this duty requires a commitment to the profession, a commitment akin to a vocation. We have to be prepared to respond to the call to work as a trustworthy nurse. To answer the call to nursing—to take the vow of nursing—is to fulfill the ethical duty of engendering trust through our practice.

Imagine the night nurse. Hungry, tired, pulled in the direction of other patients who needed her attention, the night nurse nonetheless had a commitment to her duty to respond to the young, new mother's plea. It was a plea to restore trust that had been shattered—the mother's trust in an all-natural childbirth, in breast milk untainted by drugs, in the precious moments of her newborn son suckling at her breast and, in the repose of her arms, gazing into her face as if his mother's eyes were his whole universe. It was a call—a question—to the night nurse about whether the new mother could count on her. That night nurse had a sense of the mother's shattered trust and a commitment to her duty as a nurse to build it back up—to be counted on. This commitment is to nursing not just as a job but as a calling, a vocation.

As I mentioned in Chapter 1, Frederick Beuchner has defined the notion of a vocation as an intersection between doing the work that you need most to do and the work that the world needs to have done. Without doubt, the work of nursing is among the work that the world needs to have done. Those nurses who think of their everyday, trustworthy acts of nursing practice as a commitment to restoring and promoting the public's trust have, I aver, answered the call to nursing as a vocation, something more than a job. They have found in nursing a life-calling: they must do the work of nursing because, they know, the work of nursing is good for society. This can be symbolized in what I call the vow of nursing.

In the Middle Ages, the Knights of the Hospitallers were among the first organized nurses. Commonly known as the Knights of Malta, they pinned the Cross of Malta upon the men who had taken the order's vow to care for the poor, the sick, the weary and hungry. They wore this pin on their arms to show their fidelity to this oath to all for whom they provided care. In the United States, to this day, the tradition upon graduation from nursing school is for an alum of the school to pin upon the graduate the school's "nursing pin." It is akin to taking the vow of fidelity to the order of nursing. I graduated from the Yale School of Nursing. An alumna of the school presented me with *my pin* when I graduated. The eight-pointed Cross of Malta predominates the school's pin. I wear it when I see patients. It is a symbol I wear to show patients that I have taken the profession's vow and, to the best of my ability, I will fulfill the duties of the profession I have entered. It is as if to say, "You can trust me: I am a nurse."

This comes, however, with moral responsibility. Patients and families trust that we will care for them; they give us the benefit of the doubt. When they trust us, they are giving us discretionary powers regarding the best way to do this. After all is said and done, they will judge us; and when they do, can we still say, "I am a nurse. You can trust me"?

The lore of nursing is that once a nurse, always a nurse. I have met nurses who have not practiced for years. But they still identify as nurses. There is something about the profession that means that membership does not end when one no longer practices; it extends for life. This is because the vow of providing equal access to the conditions of health and of promoting aliveness and that which sustains aliveness *is* irrevocable. The pin is a symbol of our faithfulness to our calling in making the profession of nursing our life's work. Herein lies the profession's greatest claim to trustworthiness: nurses are in the profession because it is their life's calling. They have taken a vow to care. In their everyday acts of nursing care, they prove their faithfulness—to themselves, to their patients, to their patients' communities, and to the world. This faithfulness to the vow of nursing—evidenced through their everyday habit of performing trustworthy acts of nursing care—is, I suggest, what the public means when it says that nursing is among the most trusted of the professions.

Trustworthiness is so fundamental to good nursing that it is tempting to reduce the nature of a good nurse to trustworthiness. However, this would be the same as viewing nurses as good technicians. Of course, nurses are good technicians—competent, reliable, and honest, faithful to the work at hand. But being a good nurse is more than being a competent, reliable, and honest technician. Good nursing involves an art and a wisdom beyond the technical. Good nursing involves imagination—moral imagination. It is to the habit of imagination we turn next.

Chapter 3

Imagination

We nurses are a practical tribe. We make lists for ourselves with little checkboxes beside each item. We make these checklists on almost anything: scrap pieces of paper and the back of our gloved (and sometimes bare) hands. When we tick all the checkboxes, we feel a sense of satisfaction: we know we have completed the tasks we needed to do. Our jobs demand our attention to the practical work of nursing. So it may seem odd to suggest that, amid our task-oriented daily work, developing a habit of imagination is a good thing. Wouldn't a lively imagination take us away from the work we need to get done?

The practical importance of our jobs notwithstanding, nursing and imagination do have something to do with each other. If we think about it, Henderson's definition of nursing involves imagination. Nurses, in this function, are to be the sight of the sightless, the ambulation of the maimed, the rested assurance of first-time parents, the promise of life for the suicidal, and the meaning of life for the patient newly diagnosed with cancer. In this unique function, the nurse imagines what might be sight, what might be movement, what knowledge and meaning might be, and what the future could be like for those who cannot imagine it for themselves. When we imagine our patients whole, we supply them with the fullness of humanity, even amid disease and disorder.

Most often, however, our patients do not come to us whole. They come with maladies. Sometimes, we try to imagine the misery that accompanies these maladies—the misery of our patients who are homeless, who are stricken with unquenchable addictions, and who are diagnosed with life-limiting disease. Often we say, in response to hearing our patients' miseries, "I can't even imagine!" And this is true: the experiences of another are not the same as our experiences. Even if we, too, have experienced homelessness, addiction, or serious disease, our experience of these maladies most likely differs in significant ways, if not just in our personal stories, from our patients' experiences. Can we ever truly imagine the misery of others?

Our use of imagination is not always to be trusted. I will give you two examples. First, imagining how others feel amid their maladies can lead us to take pity on them. By "pity" I mean feeling sorry for people who find themselves in circumstances we cannot imagine ourselves in. Sometimes, pity leads us to take action, such as making a donation to charity, but it does not usually propel us to address the maladies of those whom we pity. In fact, sometimes when we feel pity, we want to stay away from the people whom we pity. "I don't like going around them. Their circumstances are too dire. Being around them pulls me down," some might say. Imagining the pain of others in order to pity them is not the imagination I am talking about. I am talking about imagination that leads us to nursing action.

Second, we can, through imagination, foist our wishes upon another person. Sometimes when we see people in predicaments, we will do what we imagine they need without asking them. But what if it is not what is best for them or what they want done? In these instances, our use of imagination can become a means of pushing our wishes upon others.

However, imagination is a powerful force that we can use for good. In our unique function as nurses, we can develop the habit of imagining what our patients would do for themselves, if they had the will, knowledge, or power, to restore or promote their health or to have a peaceful death. This kind of imagination is a habit of the good nurse.

This kind of imagination—nursing imagination—involves sympathy. "Sympathy" is an old-fashioned word, nowadays most often reserved for cards to express our condolences. However, sympathy is more than a sentiment. The word, in its origins, means "feeling" (*pathy*) "together" (*syn*). This meaning of sympathy assumes a relationship—a commonality. Sympathy is, I suggest, the common feeling we share—the feeling of our humanity, the feeling of caring *for* our common humanity.

Notice that sympathy differs from empathy. "Empathy" suggests you understand or inhabit the exact feelings of another. I have already suggested that I think this is a tall, if not impossible, order. How can we know we feel the same as the other feels, given the differences of our lives? Sympathy, however, is the common feeling of caring for how others around us feel. It is the feeling of knowing what it is to care about the crying baby, the malnourished child, the abused runaway who needs shelter, the wounded accident victim. To do for patients what they would do for themselves if they could involves cultivating within ourselves the *feeling of caring* for the humanity of our patients. Our common humanity, after all, is the basis of our relationship with our patients. When we feel we care for the humanity of our patients, we imagine them in a state of health or having a peaceful death, and then we imagine the possibilities of what we can do to bridge the gap between how they are and how we imagine them to be if our care is successful. That is, sympathy is feeling the patient's desire for health or a peaceful death. It is the heart opening the mind so that we may imagine health or a peaceful death for them *and then care* for them in a way that brings this about. It is imagining a future for them *and then providing* the nursing care necessary to make that a reality. Sympathy is a feeling of care that propels us toward the work of nursing.

In a clinical situation in which life itself is compromised, we use our imaginations to see potentialities of life that we had not seen before: we are sighted, and we use our sympathetic imagination to create a world for ourselves in which we are not sighted so that we can be sight for the sightless. We deploy our imaginations as our instruments of attentiveness to life and to ways of living that we had neglected, ignored, overlooked, or never had to consider. Through sympathy we are attentive to life that is "other" to us—to our patient's life. Our unique function as nurses prompts us to use our imaginations to present the "otherness of life" to ourselves in a way that makes sense to us, in a way that we can feel the aliveness of someone who is not at all like us. Through sympathy, the "otherness of life" becomes life to us. Sympathy is an imaginative act of setting aside ourselves—our understanding of life and of the right way to live—to take on what, for others (that is, for our patients), promotes and sustains life and leads to a peaceful death for them. Sympathy is *feeling care* for the other and, in response to this feeling of care, *performing* for them the unique function of the nurse.

The aliveness of our patients may be new to us. At first it may seem as if we cannot be attentive to the aliveness of the person who is homeless, who struggles with addiction, or who is dying of a disease we are afraid of ourselves. However, imagining for our patients, regardless of who they are and what they struggle with, unleashes new possibilities within us of how to be alive and how to respond to being alive. These new possibilities awaken in us humanity we had never imagined for ourselves—the capacity to be touched by the circumstances our patients find themselves in. The capacity of being touched by the humanity of our patients is the ethical force of imagination.

Imagination, understood in this way, assumes relationship. But as nurses, this is not the mere relationship of acquaintance. It is a responsible relationship. I use the word "responsible" because our relationship with patients requires that we *respond to* them. It is the response of imagining for them a future of health or a peaceful death and acting upon that imagination. This response is a response of hope for them—our hope that their health will be promoted or restored or that their death will be peaceful. It is not so much a response to their plight of sickness or potential sickness, a response of pitying them, but rather a response to their plea to be trustworthy with their most precious gifts of their health and their hopes. To their plea for our trustworthy acts of nursing care, we respond with a vision of wholeness for them, even until death.

We see in this plea-response the nurse–patient relationship. It is not just a relationship in which the patient, by virtue of being sick or potentially sick, demands care, though it is that. It is, however, a relationship in which patients tell us their present predicament. They are potentially sick, they are sick, or they are dying. We *listen* to them in this predicament. We *listen* to what, for them, is a state of health or a peaceful death. We *listen* to their voices, to use the phrase of the great moral psychologist Carol Gilligan. Our response is, for a moment, to set aside the medical facts—lab and imaging results, hemodynamic monitoring results, electrocardiogram results, pathology results—and listen. We allow their voices, the patients' voices, to fill the room. It is their pleas, after all, that brought us into relationship with them in the first place—their pleas for our care. In listening to their voices, we hear what they hope for themselves— their imagination of what health restored or health promoted or a peaceful death would look like *for them*. It is in listening to their voice that we can imagine them before us in a restored state of health, or of safely crossing over to the other side—in the way they see it for themselves. It is their vision of the future that becomes our present imagination. And so it is not that we foist upon our patients our imagination of what their future would look like. Rather, we *respond* to their vision of a whole future. Their vision of health becomes our vision. Their vision of a peaceful death becomes our vision. It is by imagining what they would be like in their visions of themselves as whole that we can determine what they would do for themselves to achieve that vision, if they had the will, knowledge, or power. Their vision guides us in what nursing acts to undertake.

Depressed and in despair, patients may not be able to imagine a future at all. Patients are sometimes hopeless. They sometimes do not have a vision of the future. They have lost their voice. In these moments, we feel for them what they cannot feel for themselves— hope. A psychiatric nurse practitioner once told me that she has had patients who, upon their first visit with her for treatment for depression, ask her why she evaluates their depression so carefully and with such detail. She says to them, "One day, when you are better, we will look back at this first evaluation and see how far you've come." "I see a future they cannot see," she told me. "And I share that future with them." In these instances, the nurse imagines what patients would be like if they could have a vision of themselves as whole and responds to them with this vision.

The nurse–patient relationship acknowledges the patient's capacity to be equal in a relationship. To recognize this capacity is to respect the patient as fully human. "To care for a person adequately and genuinely as a person," the feminist bioethicist Margaret Farley says, "is to care for her in relation—in the context of the story of her relationships, past, present, and future." We fit into the context of our patients' stories. Our relationship with them is one among others they may have. We learn of their past and their present relationships. We fit ourselves into the story of their present relationships. And we imagine a future of relationships for them, even as they leave this life.

Sometimes we lose our relationships: our patients die. Our interventions fail, but our failure is not a failure of imagination. It is a failure of our interventions and our science. Amid these failures, however, we remain optimistic. Optimism is hoping for the best possible world to come about, even though this may be unrealistic. In this way, we nurses are optimists. Our response to our patients is hope, and the more often we respond with hope, the easier it becomes to respond imaginatively to the direst of situations.

So far we have talked about the imagination in response to our patients. It is an imagination focused not on pity toward them but, rather, on their humanity—their hopes and their fears of these hopes not coming true. We respond as fellow humans. Through imagination, we feel care for our patients. We respond to our patients' plea for assistance; we hope for them, and in hoping for them, we discover a hope we had not hitherto known, for we have not known nor heard this particular patient's plea before. Or at least, each time we hear it, we hear it anew, and we recognize in ourselves feelings of care for our fellow human.

Through our habit of imagining our patients' humanity, we find our self-knowledge as nurses. The habit of imagination is a habit of self-knowledge, of learning about ourselves through our patients. Our patients are not necessarily like us. In some instances, they are far from us, people with whom, in our normal lives, we could not identify. They are not our kith and kin. They are homeless, ill, poor, of a different gender, of a different sexuality, of a different land, of a different religion, of another language, and not our age. Their lives do not resemble ours. Yet, through imagination, we take an interest in them. They become close. We bathe them. We change their clothes and their bedding. We take their blood. We share in their joy of new life, and we break to them the sad news of impending death. They, though we do not know them, are as close to us as we are to ourselves; our humanity, after all, binds us. Our relationship with them is the wellspring of our imagining. They teach us who we can be.

We can imagine what kind of nurse we want to be. We can imagine that we want to feel care for our patients and allow this feeling to respond to our patients' pleas that we do for them what they cannot do for themselves. We can also imagine what kind of nurse we do not want to be.

The literary critic and essayist David Bromwich writes about using imagination as a way of renouncing who we do not want to be. We do not want to be a nurse who is brusque and thankless; this would be inhuman. And when we imagine who we would become if we refused to feel care for those who need it, we see someone we cannot recognize, someone inhuman. The vision of nursing is a vision of a good society—*for all*. We resist becoming the kind of nurse we do not wish to become by imagining that kind of nurse, and by imagining the kind of nurse we do not wish to become, we resist in ourselves the cruelties that detract from our being a good nurse.

I have heard about a young man who became a nurse because he saw nurses care for his brother. His brother had joined the armed forces after terrorist attacks hit the city they lived in. Sent abroad as part of a multinational force, his brother, a gunner, was riding in a convoy when his gun-truck ran over an improvised explosive device. Medics kept his brother alive in the field. A helicopter flew in, picked him up, and transported him to the field hospital. Nurses and doctors in the field hospital stitched him up as best they could and sent him home to die. At home, the nurses kept his brother comfortable, changing the dressings on his burns and making sure his pain was managed. The nurses, in somber tones, told his family when they saw the signs of impending death so that the family could sit with him in the final vigil. For this reason, the young man left his job as a clerk, went back to school, took the hard prerequisite courses (anatomy, physiology, chemistry, and biology), and then finally went to nursing school. Several years later, he was a novice nurse, full of the excitement of being able to provide technical care and in love with the very idea of nursing as a caring profession. He wanted to care as his brother had been cared for. His first job was in the emergency department (ED) of his city's largest hospital, the hospital where his brother had come home to die.

News came to his ED that there had been several explosions throughout the city. The explosions were coordinated—the hallmark of terrorism. The ED should expect large numbers of patients, the staff were told. Within minutes, the victims started rolling in, burned, maimed, and, in some cases, blown to pieces. The police accompanied one patient, however. He was not a victim; he was a suspect. He was put in one of the young man's beds. The young man saw the suspect. He saw in him the ethnicity, the tribe, the clothing, though in pieces, of the group who had killed his brother, the group that now terrorized his own country, his own city. The young man thought about it for a moment: he had the tools in his crash cart to kill this suspect. For a split second, he imagined doing it. But then he saw in his imagination the kind of person he did not want to become. He had gone into nursing, after all, not to be that inhumane person. He had gone into nursing to resist violence and terror. He became a nurse because he felt care. Unable to tolerate the image of himself as a murderous nurse, he provided the best care possible for the suspect, and he was kindhearted toward him: the nurse wiped the tears that silently fell from his patient's eyes. The young man imagined his patient, should he ever find his way back to his own people, going to his home village and telling everyone, including the leader of the terrorist sect to which he belonged, that he was cared for.

In that moment of practicing the habit of imagination, the young nurse became who he imagined himself to be: someone who felt care for the sick, someone who provided nursing care. To cultivate nursing imagination in ourselves is to feel care for others and to provide the nursing care that brings about health for the sick and a peaceful death for the dying. It is to be the kind of good nurse we want to be.

Bioethicists often speak of "capacitating" someone, that is, of making someone capable of making ethical decisions. It is in this sense that most usual nursing ethics books are written. They seek to give nurses the tools of the ethical specialist so that they can make decisions about ethically troubling problems or dilemmas in nursing practice: to unplug the ventilator of a patient in a persistent vegetative state; to deny opiates to a "drug seeker"; whether or not to tell the family behind the physician's back that their loved one really is dying, that there really is not a slim chance of recovery, as the family often is told. But these tools no more capacitate someone to maneuver these difficult waters than they teach some sort of replicable skill. There is rarely ever a clear way through the horns of these issues. Although rarely, patients have awakened from a persistent vegetative state; some patients who have opiate addictions do have untreated pain and legitimately seek relief from that pain; and sometimes patients indeed are dying when some health care providers tell loved ones that there is a slim chance of recovery. There is no one response to ethical problems and dilemmas. Principles alone cannot guide us with clarity through these treacherous waters.

Imagination, however, gives us the capacity to be touched by the circumstances of our patients and, in so doing, opens up the possibilities of a nursing response, a response that is attentive to their aliveness. It can be difficult to see the aliveness of the people for whom we care. They present to us scarred by disease and disorder, decaying from the dying process, or as the worried well, people merely bothered by the vagaries of life. But our patients present to us for nursing care because they are alive and they want to remain alive and because they want to enhance their aliveness, however they may find themselves at present. We need to cultivate in ourselves the ability to see the aliveness of our patients, to see the beauty in being alive. As we will see in the next chapter, it is through what I call the "habit of beauty" that our nursing care takes on a different dimension, the dimension of bringing justice to our patients' injuries.

Chapter 4

Beauty

I will leave this earth with the memory of this event. It was horrible, so horrible, in fact, its repulsiveness is forever etched in my mind—indelibly etched, etched with the acid of injustice. Even now, I can conjure up the moment it happened; and even now, I feel its injury. I say "the moment it happened" because it was one of those moments in which the event isolated itself, set itself off from everything else. It was the only event in my consciousness at the time. Everything else going on disappeared, even my awareness of being in my body. Darkness took over everything. It was so horrible.

I was abroad. Three graduate students were with me as research assistants. They were in their mid-twenties, all quite mature and dedicated to advanced practice nursing. We were standing in the middle of a hospital ward. We had been in this ward daily for almost a month collecting data on symptoms from patients. We knew that one of the patients on the ward was near death. We had seen her before. We knew her clinical situation. She was in quite a lot of pain; this she had told us, but her body told as much, too. She writhed in bed. We tried to get the physicians on the ward to give her pain medication. Fear of using opiates and lack of opiate supply conspired; her pain remained unmanaged for the month we had been on the ward.

As we stood there that morning, a crisp, bright morning, the sun's rays entered the ward's windows and danced on the bare cement floor. We had arrived early so that we could start collecting data just after the physicians finished rounding. The ward buzzed; it was crowded with patients in beds and with patients who were not hospitalized but who were waiting to see the physicians after they finished rounding. That morning the ward buzzed, and it rocked with this patient's moans. We stood there, the four of us, in the middle of the ward, waiting to collect data from patients. We remarked to each other that this woman's moans were different this morning, this bright morning, this morning full of the buzzing business of the ward.

As her moans grew into shrieks, I looked in her direction. A family member stood by her side. Two nurses attended her. They were washing her limbs and brow with cool cloths, the pain management techniques they had available to them. Her shrieks turned to screams, screams like I had never known before. We know the death rattle; its sound is familiar to us. It is the sound of secretions piling up in the throat and upper chest, which dying patients cannot clear. I knew the death rattle. But I had not known the death scream, not until I heard it that morning. My students heard it, too. We heard this woman scream the death scream, and in the very middle of that scream, she died. She announced her death with that scream, and then she died. The scream, loud and desperate, shook everything— our bones, our minds, our hearts.

It was sad, gut-wrenching, depressing, unfathomable. It was all that. But more than all that, it was violent, repulsive, unjust. Its injustice disturbed me, disturbed me as far down as I could be disturbed. It was one of the most horrible events I have ever experienced—a dying woman screaming into her death.

"Beauty," Augustine said, is "a plank amid the waves of the sea." The sea waves that morning on the ward—dark and cold and rogue—overtook this woman; and in the moment, they overtook us. As soon as we came to our senses, my students and I stepped outside into the hospital's garden. The sun was warm and strong. We stood by a tree; it had the most beautiful red blossoms on it. Bougainvillea with purple flowers climbed up trellises on the hospital's walls; they, too, were beautiful. We saw the beauty of these flowers, of their colors and shapes; and we felt the sun hitting our backs, taking the edge off the coldness that had settled into our bones. Beauty was the saving plank amid the waves of the stormy sea that morning.

Daily we nurses sail on stormy seas, and daily we need the saving plank of beauty. The hospital's gardens were beautiful, exotically beautiful—nature's beauty. "Beauty," the essayist Elaine Scarry says, "is lifesaving." But the beauty that preserved me amid that dark and choppy sea that morning was not the beauty of the gardens or the warm sun. What saved me that morning was the beauty of nursing. The nurses themselves and their nursing acts aimed at alleviating the dying woman's pain were beauty, beauty amid the injuries of pain.

Injury, not ugliness, is the opposite of beauty. In fact, the base of the word "injury," Scarry points out, is *jur*, which means right, right in the sense of justice. An injury is an event that is not right. An injury is an injustice. To die a death that is not peaceful is an injustice; it is not right. The nurses who attended the dying woman, in their healing acts of addressing her pain with the only tools they had, addressed the pain that injured the dying woman's humanity.

It is in this sense that injury is wrong—morally wrong: injury threatens life. There are public health injuries that threaten life— lead-laced water the public have been told is safe to drink, the Earth that is warming up to degrees unsustainable for life, inadequate resources to address diseases and pain and suffering equally around the world. And there are personal injuries that threaten life. Nursing practice, in its unique function, addresses these injuries. Nursing practice, by addressing these injuries, seeks to beget beauty, and beauty is life-saving.

Beauty is life-saving to patients through the work of nurses. Nurses, Annie Goodrich says, should have a "love of beauty," for beauty motivates nurses to restore and promote health and to lead patients to serene deaths. But for this to be the case, nurses need to develop the habit of seeing their patients as beautiful. It is not so much that our patients are beautiful in the sense of a supermodel or someone whose physical presence matches that of Michelangelo's David. We often see patients in their injured state. Even if they look like a Gisele or an Adonis, they come to us injured or potentially injured. Our choice as nurses is to imagine the beauty of their lives.

Let me illustrate with an example from my own practice. I assumed the care of a patient in an oncology clinic because the nurse practitioner who had been caring for him went out on leave. The patient had prostate cancer, but it was not clear if the cancer had spread or was contained in the prostate. The patient, a man about a decade older than me, struggled with anxiety. It debilitated him at times, leaving him alone in his home, shut off from daily life. Even to come to the hospital to see me, he would have to take anti-anxiety medication. Unemployed, he always came to appointments with his partner, a woman of about his age who worked but whose job did not bring in much money. She was loving and attentive: she took notes on everything I said during the appointments and repeated them back to me to make sure she understood my instructions. They both wanted his prostate cancer treated. But there was an obstacle that was getting in the way.

The oncologist wanted my patient to have a colonoscopy to screen for colon cancer before he would make a decision about how to treat the tumor in the patient's prostate. This is common. We need as much information as possible when making treatment decisions about cancer care. But going under the sedation necessary for a colonoscopy frightened my patient. He had been refusing this colonoscopy for several months before I become involved in his care. Although no one called him "a problem patient," some clinicians who had worked with him hinted that he was. And I admit, a few times I found myself impatient with him, he was so full of anxiety. One day, he and his partner came to the clinic to see me. It was a winter day, and the heat was on a bit too high in the clinic room. One of them had been smoking cigarettes; though my patient said he did not smoke, the room reeked when I entered it. The overpowering smell, the heat, and my frustration at my patient's refusal to have a colonoscopy—yet again—got the best of me. I started to feel physically ill. In the middle of that visit, I thought I had come to my end. I did not think I could care for my patient anymore.

The choice I had in that moment was how I viewed my patient. I knew it would be two weeks before I saw him again, so I had two weeks to start imagining a future for him. I started telling myself a story about him in my head. I knew a bit about his life; I had, after all, taken his social history. I knew where he was born and raised, how much education he had had, and what he used to do for work. I knew that anxiety debilitated him, and I knew that his mother, who had died of cancer, was also "an anxious sort." His father had passed away, too; this I knew. I knew enough to start imagining my patient as other than a "prostate cancer patient" in my clinic room. I started imagining him as having lived a life before my life with him. I also started imagining him as having a life with a future, a future of getting a colonoscopy and of getting the right treatment for the prostate tumor. And I imagined a future for him in which he did not come again to the cancer clinic, a future in which he did not need to come because the cancer had been controlled. I hoped for a future for him free from disease.

This is our choice as nurses—the choice to view our patients as having lives outside the context in which we see them. It is an ethical choice. It is the choice to view our patients as if disease and disorder do not rule their lives, even though they may be afflicted with disease and beset by disorder. It is the choice of viewing our patients as having beautiful lives. Life, after all, is beautiful.

Stories—our patients' stories, how we interact with our patients' stories, and the stories we tell ourselves about patients, as I did with my anxious oncology patient—have the power to transform how we view our patients.

I recently went to the Neue Galerie in New York City with my wife. She wanted to see Gustav Klimt's *Portrait of Adele Bloch-Bauer*. I didn't care to see it. I am not a big fan of Klimt's work; it doesn't resonate with me. But my wife wanted to see it. About a month before, she had seen the movie *Woman in Gold*, about Klimt's portrait of Bloch-Bauer. Since then, she was on a mission to see the actual portrait. It was a very cold and windy late December morning that I found myself waiting in line with my wife to get into the gallery to see the "Woman in Gold" portrait. We waited for an hour. The movie had made it one of the most popular paintings to see in New York City. We finally got into the gallery, walked upstairs, and saw the portrait. After a few minutes of looking at it, I was done. My opinion of Klimt's work had not changed. But my wife kept looking at the painting. She circled around the room and looked at it from seemingly all possible angles. She walked into a different room and looked at different pieces of art and then went back into the room in which the "Woman in Gold" hangs. She looked at it again and again. I was stupefied about what captured her attention. After we left the gallery, she said it was so beautiful, so breathtakingly beautiful. I asked her what was beautiful about it; I just didn't see what captured her so much. She said, "Oh, you don't know the story. You need to watch the movie."

A few days later, I watched the movie, *Woman in Gold*, which tells the story of Maria Altmann trying to reclaim Klimt's *Portrait of Adele Bloch-Bauer*, who was Altmann's aunt. When Altmann was young, in the years before World War II, she lived in Vienna in the same house as her aunt. They had a very close relationship. Altmann, who was Jewish and from a wealthy family, fled Vienna just as the Nazis were about to detain her. Her escape was daring, as the movie portrayed, so daring that as I watched the movie, I grew anxious that Altmann would get caught and be sent to the concentration camps. But she escaped. Eventually, she made her way to the United States, where she lived the remainder of her life. During her life in the United States, she often remembered the portrait Klimt painted of her aunt, the portrait that graced her childhood Viennese home. But the Nazis stole the portrait, and after the war, the Austrian government claimed the portrait belonged to the country, not to Altmann, Bloch-Bauer's sole surviving heir. Altmann, who in her later life in the United States was a woman of modest means, spent years trying to recover the Klimt portrait of her aunt. This was Altmann's story: a story of her being a refugee, a story of the Nazis killing her family, a story of her family's history ripped off the walls of their house and then reappropriated by the Nazis and the Austrian government, and a story of struggle to regain that which was rightfully hers. After years of struggle, the Austrian government returned the Klimt portrait to Maria Altmann; and now, it hangs in the Neue Galerie in New York City, where Altmann, now deceased, wanted it to hang.

After I watched the movie, my wife said to me, "See why the portrait is so beautiful?" The story—the awful but amazing story—transformed what I had seen with my eyes into something more. It was more than a mere portrait painted by Klimt. It was the whole story, a story of unspeakable injustice that ended with the triumph of justice. And so it is with our patients. They may come to us anxious. They may be what other clinicians have labeled them— "uncompliant" or "patient does not adhere to treatment plan of getting a screening colonoscopy." They may come to us with all kinds of diseases and disorders, injustices beyond their control. But their human story transforms our opinions of these unbeautiful aspects of their lives into something beautiful.

I now think of my time in the presence of that Klimt portrait as a time in which I was in the presence of something transcendent, something that inspires awe. I now can think of that portrait as awe-inspiring. Its story transformed my view of it. I now choose to see the portrait as beautiful, and with that choice, the portrait bestows upon me a sense of awe.

Awe, the philosopher Immanuel Kant suggested, is associated with morality. There was something good (in the sense of moral) about the story of how Klimt's portrait now hangs in the gallery Maria Altmann chose for it. There is something good about restitution, about Altmann's relentless struggle for restitution—for justice. This struggle inspired in me a feeling of awe. I haven't gone back to see the portrait again, but even now, the memory I have of standing in its presence is transformed by knowing its story. I feel awe at its beauty, the beauty the story bestowed upon it. Our patients' stories bestow beauty upon them, and we can choose to stand in their presence with a sense of awe.

When we view our patients as beautiful, their beauty, not the disease and disorder that injures them, fills our minds. Our minds, then, full of beauty, search for something beyond our patients in order to fit them into a larger scene, the *mise en scène* of all the beautiful things of their lives—even the beauty of life itself. It is a moment of life untrammeled by the injuries of disease and disorder. When we choose to see our patients as beautiful, we see them in the fullness of their lives, their lives as if they were not beset with injustices. We stand in their presence with a sense of awe—awe that they are here, awe that they are alive. When we do this, we engage in an imaginative exercise that creates life for them. Through our decision to look upon our patients as beautiful, we create the beauty of our patients' present lives—beauty amid pain and suffering and disease and disorder.

And so it was with my patient who was too anxious to get a colonoscopy. The next time I saw him, I had a new attitude toward him, an attitude in which I thought of his life as beautiful. And I stood in awe of him, at his being alive, at his wanting to do what he needed to do to stay alive. He may have been too anxious to undergo the sedation necessary to get a colonoscopy, but he wanted to be alive. He kept all his appointments with me, after all; he was doing the best he could. I told him so. Well, I didn't tell him that he was beautiful, but I did say that I cared for him and wanted to do whatever he needed me to do so that he could get the colonoscopy. He said he would get the colonoscopy if I went with him. I did; it was a struggle to schedule so that I could go, but I did. We booked the appointment for the procedure. When the day came I met him and his partner at the procedure clinic. I had told the nurse anesthetist ahead of time about my patient's anxiety, and she and I came up with a plan about what anti-anxiety medication he could take before coming. Even with this medication in his system, he was still anxious. The anesthetist came out to the waiting room and walked with my patient into the procedure room and properly sedated him. He did it. He underwent the sedation necessary and got the colonoscopy. In the end, he didn't have any polyps. After the procedure, he began treatment for his prostate cancer. His regular nurse practitioner came back from leave, and I have never seen this man again. But I do remember him not so much as an anxious man but as a man who was doing what he could to stay alive.

The intentional choice of viewing our patients as beautiful is a choice of leaning toward justice. When we look upon our patients as beautiful, we choose to believe that all patients have the same right to have their injustices redressed. We feel within ourselves the demand to redress their injustices with our everyday, trustworthy acts of nursing care. In fact, it is our nursing care that aims to right our patients' injustices. Acts of nursing care seek to right the injustices that threaten our patients' beauty. When we look upon our patients as beautiful, when we see all who need nursing care as beautiful, we transform our thinking in such a way that we see our patients as having the right to have their injustices addressed—whether by restoring or promoting their health or providing them a serene death. Beauty addresses injustice. As Goodrich says, we nurses have a love of beauty; and because of this, we address our patients' injustices.

We can choose to see our patients, in the fullness of their human stories, as beautiful. When we do, we create a moment in our patients' lives when they are free from injury: we see them as fully alive. In so doing, we bring life to them; we give them the fullness of their lives. When we decide to view our patients as beautiful, we stand before the fullness of their lives with a sense of awe. We vow to do for them what they would do, if they had the will, knowledge, or power, to bring themselves back to the fullness of life, even as cancer threatens it or even as they lay dying in pain. Our seemingly most mundane acts of nursing care become sublime—giving a bed bath, changing the bed, holding a spoonful of ice chips up to parched lips, sitting silently by the bed and holding the hand of the dying. Through our decision to look upon our patients as beautiful, these acts become more than merely life-saving: they become life-giving.

Our seemingly mundane acts of nursing care bestow upon our patients that which is justly theirs—life, even as they are dying.

It is as if when we come to our patients to perform our every-day, trustworthy acts of nursing care, we knock at the doors of their lives and present to them a gift, the gift of our care, the gift of look-ing upon them as beautiful human beings worthy of our care. It is only when we do this that our patients welcome us into their lives. "Welcome" means that we come into our patients' lives—that we become part of their life stories—with their consent. Our patients, when they welcome us into their lives, consent to our request to be part of their lives. And that is just what looking upon our patients as beautiful is: a request to be part of the healing of their lives, the restoration or the promotion of their lives to health or to aid them in achieving a peaceful death. It is only when we choose to see the beauty of our patients that they can say to us, "I know that you're here for my good. I can see this by how you look upon me. And so, I welcome you. I present to you my consent for you to work on my body and mind. I present to you my well wishes for you to care for me." This welcome is our patients' response to our choice of think-ing about them as beautiful.

This notion of welcome is inherent in Henderson's definition of nursing. Through beholding the patient as beautiful, the nurse wel-comes the patient into the common place where their wills become one regarding the nursing care necessary to restore or promote health or to lead to a peaceful death. In this aligning of each oth-er's wills regarding the nursing care necessary, the nurse's strength and knowledge become one with the patient's. In the same essay in which she describes her concept of nursing, Henderson credits Goodrich with the centrality of the ethics inherent in it. And indeed, the notion of welcome in Henderson's definition is part and parcel of the habit of beauty.

There are times when our patients do not welcome us into their lives, even though we come with the good intentions of bestowing upon them the abundance of aliveness. In some instances, we can still protect them from disease and disorder if we think they are likely to harm themselves or others. But when patients do not welcome us, we still can choose to look upon them as beautiful. We still can choose to see them as alive human beings. We can still try to see their beauty.

At first, I could not see it, when the woman died amid her screams. I could not see beauty. I stood alive; she lay dead. It took some time and some soul-searching. It was like seeing Klimt's portrait of Bloch-Bauer. I needed to reframe the story; I needed to decide to find the beauty in the woman's story. Those two nurses, doing what they could do to relieve the dying woman's pain, pain that was surely physical but probably also emotional and spiritual, chose to see the beauty in the patient's life, even as she lay dying. They chose to set aside their anger at the system, their distress at the health care providers who would not prescribe enough pain medications; they chose to set all that aside and see the patient as beautiful and to meet the demands of her beauty. Beauty demanded they act to relieve her pain as best they could. Beauty demanded they act for her good.

Our patients do not share fully in life when they are sick or potentially sick or dying. We recognize that, and as nurses, we are called upon by the moral character of our profession to right it—to make it just. We engage in acts of nursing practice that bring life to our patients, acts that bring justice to their injuries. Because our patients, by virtue of being patients, do not participate equally in life, we act to balance the scales of justice. In this balancing, the focus is on our patients, not on ourselves. Our patients become the center of our thoughts and our actions. Taking ourselves out of the center is an act of "unselfing," as the writer and philosopher Iris Murdoch called it. "Unselfing" is the act of creating the space in our hearts and minds and our actions for the aliveness of our patients. We no longer focus on how difficult our jobs are with "uncompliant" patients, patients who do not "adhere to our treatment plan." When we "unself," we open up the space in ourselves for our patients' lives and the stories of their lives. "Unselfing," through our conscious choice, brings our patients into the center of our field of vision. What we then see is their beauty, as if they were the portrait hanging in the art museum. That is, decentering ourselves—"unselfing" ourselves—distributes beauty to our patients. We are, in effect, saying that they are beautiful human beings who deserve all that beauty demands. When we perform our everyday, trustworthy acts of nursing practice, we answer the demands of beauty. Answering the demands of beauty is an act of justice, and we bring justice to the injuries of our patients' lives.

I now see my viewing Klimt's *Portrait of Adele Bloch-Bauer* as an act of answering the demands of beauty. I now see the portrait as beautiful because of its story, the story of the Nazis' injury to Maria Altmann and her family and the long story of justice: it now hangs where its rightful owner wanted it to hang. This is a beautiful story of justice. In the same way, I can now see how those two nurses brought justice to that dying woman. By applying cool compresses to her, those two nurses were doing all they could to right the scales of justice. They took themselves out of the center; their patient became the only thing they thought about, the only thing they saw. Maybe they did what I did with my patient: maybe they imagined her life. Maybe she was a mother. Most certainly she was a daughter. She had had an ordinary life at one time, and maybe they imagined her in that ordinary life, even if they did not know anything about it. But by imagining her as a woman with a life, they saw her as alive and bore witness to her aliveness. And then they knew they had to do whatever they could to attend to—to bear witness to—her aliveness. They treated her as a beautifully alive human being. They affirmed her aliveness.

This is a fundamental truth we cannot escape: we all share the human story, and that story is beautiful. Beauty is the beginning of the human story, and beauty—the beauty of the life that was lived—is the happy ending. We have to believe our patients have a story and that, as nurses, we share that story. As nurses, our place in the beautiful story of life is a place of justice. The beauty of nursing is that nursing addresses the injustices of disease and disorder. Nursing's work is to restore justice, the justice beauty demands.

Chapter 5

Space

Patients present to us in the clinic, the hospital, the Ebola ward, the accident scene. They present to us sick, potentially sick, or dying; and insofar as they are sick, potentially sick, or dying, they are vulnerable. We write in our notes "Patient presents with," and then we write their chief complaint. Yet they present to us not merely to have their complaint addressed. They present to us to lessen their vulnerability. Laboring mothers present to us to reduce the chances that something will go wrong with them or their babies. Well patients present to us so that we can promote their health and prevent potential diseases; they present to us so that we can help them live a long and healthy life. Sick patients present to us to treat their diseases and disorders, accident victims to repair their injuries, and dying patients to lessen their suffering.

The places our patients present to us are, for the most part, industrial places, places constructed for conducting the work of health care: hospitals, clinics, skilled nursing facilities, schools, and birthing centers. Sometimes they present to us in ambulances or on the roadside at the scene of an accident. These are noisy places, busy places, places constructed for function, not for aesthetics. They are public places where privacy is lost in the pursuit of treating the body. We try to preserve physical privacy in these public places. Yet flimsy gowns, often paper, cover very little of their bodies. Examining rooms have doors that open to halls, from which, when the rooms' doors open, passersby can see patients sitting on the examining tables on thin sheets of tissue paper that separate their naked backsides from cold examining tables. Patients cohabit in hospital rooms in which the roommate and the roommate's visitors can see the tubes put into patients' bodies and the fluids coming out. We hold conversations behind drawn curtains in which loved ones must make decisions about life and death, and though we speak in hushed tones, patients and families in adjacent beds can hear everything we say. Our patients present to us in these public spaces of business in sick or potentially sick bodies, with sick or potentially sick minds, with broken hearts and downcast spirits, thinking (hoping, praying) that all is well when all is not—and sometimes, they present to us dying. They present to us in the height of their lives, vital and strong, with children at home and careers in full bloom, because they have a cold that will not go away—a mere cold—that turns out to be lymphoma. Whoever they are and for whatever reasons they present to us, they present to us to lessen their vulnerability.

When patients present to us in their vulnerability, they, by virtue of their presentation, resist vulnerability. They resist unsafe births, disease, and death. From within their vulnerabilities, they resist vulnerability. The suicidal patient calling the helpline resists suicide. The mother who cannot get her newborn to latch on to the breast and cries to the nurse-midwife for help resists despair. The patient with newly diagnosed advanced cancer who asks for "all the guns to be pulled out" resists the equation of cancer with death. Our patients, though vulnerable, present to us because they believe that our nursing care is part of their resisting vulnerability. They are, after all, reliant on our care to make them whole, to keep them whole, or to help them die well. By virtue of their presenting to us, they are in relationship with us.

Relationships are, to use the hackneyed phrase, two-way streets. In the nurse–patient relationship, patients have already walked down the street toward us. In fact, their presentation to us initiated our relationship with them. Our response to their presentation creates the space of care in the public places of health care and in the heart of patients' vulnerability. This is the fourth habit of a good nurse: creating the space of care.

In Chapter 2, I suggested that sympathy leads us to respond imaginatively to our patients' vulnerability. When we see our patients' vulnerability, we feel concern for them. This feeling is our human response to our patients' human needs. This is sympathy, and we must use it to ignite our compassion. Compassion is often the reason many of us became nurses. A nurse responded to us with compassion in our moment of need. It is why I became a nurse.

My mother was dying of advanced cancer. She was in the intensive care unit, septic and unconscious. My siblings and I had to make a decision about her care—do we put her on life support and try to fight the infection, or do we move her to hospice so that she can die without machines involved? We were not clinicians; we did not understand health care. We were given technical medical information, but it did not make sense. We did not know what to do. We had meetings with clinicians, but they did not help us maneuver through the narrow straits. This was our mother, after all; we wanted to do what was right. This had been going on for a full two days, and our distress seemed to grow by the hour. One of my mother's nurses sensed our distress. She asked if she could meet with us. We gathered around my mother's bed in the open place of the intensive care unit. The nurse pulled the curtain, and she asked us to tell her about our mother. We told her our stories. We recalled how she was a taskmaster with us about practicing the piano, how she would dress up on Halloween and frighten us, how she was a progressive woman, how she would never give up—on anything—and how she loved us. This nurse listened, and in her listening, we felt her compassion. She showed concern for us, and in that moment of her response to us, she opened a space for us—a space in the public place of the industrial intensive care unit—in which we could be ourselves and make a decision that matched who we knew our mother to be.

We nurses open up the space of care by our compassionate response to patients and families. Yet compassion without action is not useful. If we feel compassion for patients and families and do not act, we merely add pity to pain and distress. Nursing care is the form that compassion takes when we respond to patients and families who present to us in need. That is, compassion compels us to care. When we answer compassion's call to care for the injured, the oppressed, the person in pain, the person not whole, or the distressed family, we create a space for patients and families to inhabit in which they can, through our acts of nursing care, resist disease, disorder, or untimely deaths.

When we care, we take concrete actions that restore or promote health or that lead to peaceful deaths. We care for our patients and families with competent, reliable, and honest acts of nursing practice. We care for them by imagining what they would do for themselves if they had the will, knowledge, or power. We care for them by gazing upon them as beautiful—a just gaze that distributes aliveness equally to them and to us. As we care for them, we resist their vulnerability along with them.

My mother was vulnerable. Death was nigh. My siblings and I knew it. Yet we did not want to shorten her life. Maybe she could come back and spend a few more months with us. That nurse, whose name I still do not know, understood that. Through her nursing care, she invited us to see our mother as alive, to see her as the strong mother on whom, when we were young, we depended for our very lives. Through this nurse's act of compassionate nursing care, she resisted my mother's vulnerability. She did for my mother what my mother could not do for herself. She did it for us, too. We were vulnerable to the system, but that nurse resisted our vulnerability by taking us out of the system, if only for a moment, and giving us the space to be a family.

As I touched on in Chapter 2, we nurses are in a responsible relationship with our patients and their families. We feel the weight of that responsibility. We chart detailed notes to make sure the health care team knows what we did—that we delivered the right nursing care. The importance of delivering competent, evidence-based nursing care notwithstanding, it is not the basis for our responsible relationship with patients and families. The basis is compassionate care. When we respond to patients and families with compassionate care, we go toward them on the two-way street; and when we meet each other, something extraordinary happens. In the public and sterile places of the industrial health care complex, our coming together creates a space for patients and families to be who they are. Who they are—not who they present to us as.

Patients and families can be themselves in this space we have made. They present to us as vulnerable, but in the context of the space we create, we see something other than their vulnerability. We see a future of health and wholeness and peacefulness as they pass. We project into the space of care that which they need. When we do this, we create, amid the impersonal, public places of health care, a space of hope, a space for healing.

Consider Alexis's story. Alexis grew up in a small village, where her immigrant parents, devout in their faith, raised her as a boy, her biological sex. In primary school, she dressed in her mother's traditional clothes and paraded in front of the mirror, looking at herself with satisfaction. It was fun, and her mother took great joy in it, too. During adolescence, however, her father stopped her from cross-dressing and made her try out for boys' sports, at which she failed miserably. She excelled academically, especially at mathematics; but her father wanted her to be an athletic boy. Both her brothers (one older, the other younger) played sports every season of the year. Her father stopped being interested in Alexis, showering his affections on his other two sons. Later in her life, Alexis recounted her middle school years as an "era of confusion," unsure whether she was a boy or a girl; and although she saw both of her brothers with girlfriends, she felt asexual. Confusion led to depression.

In secondary school, she started self-mutilating, which led to hospitalizations and rounds of antipsychotic medications. Her once-bright mind dulled. Her father, who owned a pharmacy, stopped speaking to her. One night, a particularly low night when she had started cutting again, she overheard her father saying to her mother that the family had an image to keep up in the village and among the people with whom they worshipped. Alexis was ruining that image. "What would everyone think and say!" He said to her mother, "Either he grows up to be a good lad, or he's out of my house." That night, Alexis ran away from home, just a few months away from finishing secondary school.

She ended up in the largest city of her country. After living in and out of homeless shelters, she found a group of transgender and transsexual, or trans*, friends. They lived together in abandoned buildings, in shelters, in flats they rented by the week, when they could afford them. They made whatever living they could through sex work. In this city, Alexis was known only as Alexis. She always dressed as a woman, spoke as a woman, walked as a woman. In fact, among her group of trans* friends, she was the best-looking woman, receiving more catcalls from construction workers than any of them. She was gorgeous, young, and lithe. She looked like a runway model. Even though her life was hard and she felt anchorless, this was, she said, the happiest time of her life.

A social worker at the shelter for lesbian, gay, bisexual, and transgender youth she was living in at the time told her about a free clinic. The social worker encouraged her to go so that she could be screened for human immunodeficiency virus (HIV), and if she were still HIV-negative, she could apply to be part of a program to receive preexposure prophylaxis for free. Alexis went to the clinic. At the front desk, the receptionist took Alexis's government-issued identification card. On it was her legal name, a typical male name and a name that, to almost anyone, identified her parents' land of origin and religion. Alexis said to the receptionist, "Please call me Alexis. Please." The receptionist wrote this on the chart. Minutes later, however, a nurse stood in the doorway between the clinic area and the waiting room. Projecting her voice loud enough to be heard throughout the waiting room, she called Alexis's birth name. A man in the room, who looked as if he was from Alexis's parents' land of origin, looked up at her. Not just did everyone know, at that very moment, that Alexis was a transgender woman but this man knew even more than that. He knew Alexis's ethnicity and the religion in which she was raised. This man stood up in the waiting room and started calling Alexis names and threatening her life.

Alexis left the clinic without seeing anyone. She ran, quite literally, back to the shelter and told the social worker what had happened. The social worker tried to calm Alexis down and reassure her, but Alexis was inconsolable. Alexis left the shelter. No one has seen her since, the staff say. No one knows where she is or what has happened to her.

In what appear to be insignificant ways, our patients present to us. Their presentation to us is an act of resisting vulnerability. They present to us: "Here am I, I am Alexis." In this presentation, they ask us to respond as nurses whom they can trust—as nurses who will imagine a future for them in which they are whole, as nurses who will redress their injuries, distributing to them the justice beauty deserves. "Here am I, I am Alexis" was an act of presentation that pleaded, "Meet me where I am. Help me resist my vulnerability."

In Alexis's case, the clinic staff did not respond with compassionate care. The space of care did not result. Instead, she was met with the structures of the industrial health care complex, the public place of the clinic in which the rules of calling people by the names on their government-issued identification prevail. In the clinic, there was no space for Alexis.

We nurses share in the human condition. We are vulnerable, too. We are vulnerable to disease and disorder, and we become patients. We see our primary care providers for health promotion and prevention. Diseases visit us, and so do the effects of disorders, including accidents and natural disasters that imperil health. We will one day most certainly die, and as with our patients and their families, we want a gentle and painless death. We need nursing care just as anyone else does. What makes the space of care we create with our patients and their families more powerful—and more real—is that, in this space, we appear not only as nurses who act to lessen our patients' and their families' vulnerability but also as humans who are vulnerable to disease, disorder, and death. It is in our moments of being aware of our humanity that we gain insight into the importance of being harbingers of wholeness.

That is exactly what that nurse did for my siblings and me—and for our mother. Although a nurse acting in her nursing role, she met us as fully human. And she listened to us as we told my mother's story. In the telling of it, we understood what we needed to do and what our mother needed from us. That day, I heard in that nurse's humanity a voice that called me to care for the sick and their families in the way she had. Experiencing her compassionate nursing care was, quite literally, a moment that changed my life. I knew that I had to become a nurse. In the space of care this nurse created for us, my siblings and I found a genuineness, an authenticity: we could see our mother's humanity, and we felt our own. The loudness of the machines of the intensive care unit and the demand to make decisions about issues beyond our ken fell away. In the space of care, we found the strength to resist our mother's and our vulnerability. We became our strongest, most authentic selves. That is the power of the space of care—to restore that part of ourselves that vulnerability has stripped away.

I did not know Alexis. Yet I can imagine that Alexis had a rough edge. Her life, after all, had been rough. I can also imagine that she let few people into her life, for the people she had loved had shunned her. She was alone and struggling. She was vulnerable to HIV. I understand the clinic had to follow rules. However, she presented not just as someone who was resisting her vulnerability but as who she was: "Call me Alexis." This request encapsulated the whole of her story—her years of struggle, her years of being an outcast, and now, her attempt at becoming whole. In her request, we hear her plea that, even though she was entering the industrial health care complex, we create the space for her to be herself, a human vulnerable to disease but a human full of hope for a future of health. We can create the space for our patients to be who they truly are by responding to their pleas with compassionate nursing care. This is the habit of a good nurse.

Chapter 6

Presence

Nursing is a busy job. In the clinic, we see patient after patient, with no time in between. In the hospital, we have too many patients, and they are sick—very sick. In the home, we are conscious of whom we have to see next, when we have to be there, and how long it will take us to get there. No matter where we take care of patients, we are backlogged on charting; indeed, charting seems to take the most time of all. Our work is nonstop. This is the reality of nursing.

I have rarely ever met a nurse who has not sighed at the unrelenting busyness of our work. There is in our sigh an ardent appeal for why we are nurses. We are nurses to take care of people, and the busyness of our work seems to get in the way of that. Maybe you are a nurse because a nurse took care of you, as the nurse in the intensive care unit took care of my siblings and me. Maybe someone in your family was a nurse and you wanted to be like her or him. For whatever reason you became a nurse, now that you are one, the reason for remaining a nurse is to take care of people.

Taking care of people involves the technical aspects of evidence-based nursing practice. To be sure, good nurses practice with the best of skills and as the evidence suggests. Yet taking care of people requires more than technical skills and following evidence-based algorithms. Taking care of people requires presence.

You may have had the experience of talking with someone, and, at some point in the conversation, realizing that the person with whom you were talking, though looking straight at you, was not listening. Of course, we all have sat in a lecture and, well into the lecture, realized that we have not heard a word; we "zoned out." Likewise, we can "zone out" while nursing. The technical aspects of nursing practice can cause us to "zone out" from the prime reason we are nurses—to take care of the person who is our patient.

Whether we are working around a patient's bed, adjusting settings on an IV machine, listening to a patient's heart sounds, or drawing blood for labs, we are in the presence of a person. It is true, our patients have bodies; and it is on these bodies that we often work. They also have thoughts and emotions. We work with them on these aspects of their lives as well. More than mere bodies or mere minds, our patients have complex lives. They have stories, the stories of their lives but also the stories about why they are now our patients. When we nurse, we are in the presence of people whose stories dwell in their bodies and their minds. As nurses, we need to practice the awareness that we are not caring for a patient with a physical or mental ailment. The people we care for are not simply schizophrenic patients, cancer patients, heart patients, diabetes patients, maternity patients, or primary care patients. Rather, they are people who are sick or potentially sick. Said even more simply, we care for people. The habit I wish to speak about now is the awareness that we are in the presence of a person when we are nursing.

Have you ever taken a seat on a plane and wondered who the stranger is sitting next to you? What makes turbulence on a flight an intimate moment with that stranger is the thought of dying together, should the plane go down. Who is this stranger with whom I may share my last breath? In this moment, we realize the stranger is not a stranger; the stranger is a person, a person who has lived a life, who has loved ones, who has had happy moments and moments of disappointment, a person with a story just as we have stories. So it is with our patients. We share intimate moments with them, moments when we wash their bodies and brush their teeth, moments when we examine their most private parts, moments when we hold their newborn babies, cool their fevered brows, and hold their hands as they pass. In these moments, we provide nursing care to people, people whom we may know but people who are, most likely, strangers. Whether or not we know the stories of our patients' lives, we as nurses are in the presence of people when we provide nursing care.

In the moment of turbulence on the plane, we encounter in the stranger sitting next to us the reality of our common humanity. She or he is a person like me. To be in the presence of a person is to find "a location in human experience" where we "encounter the reality of ourselves and others," writes the feminist bioethicist Margaret Farley. To be in the presence of a person is to see the other as having the same vulnerabilities, the same hopes for a good life, and the same fears of suffering as we have. It is to gain access to a concrete reality that is deeper than the technical tasks of nursing care. We gain access to the reality of the person who is our patient.

To acknowledge personhood, the very least we must do is to respect another's capacity to make decisions and, as we saw in Chapter 3, to be in relationships. This is why we seek our patient's consent before we undertake any act of nursing care: our patient has the capacity for free choice; if we abridge this capacity, we make the patient into something less than a person. Our nursing care is not truly care unless we respect the person's right to accept or reject it. If we foist our care upon a patient, we have abridged her or his capacity (and right) to decide what is done to her of him. To recognize that we are in the presence of a person is to respect that we are in the presence of someone who has the capacity for controlling what is done to her or him.

Equally, as previously discussed, we must respect that a person has the capacity to be in relationship. This is the capacity to know and to love and to be known and to be loved. That is, a person has concrete relationships in the here and now. A person knows and loves other people. A person knows and loves a dog, a cat, a horse. A person knows and loves nature. And a person is known and loved by others. A person has loved ones with whom she or he has relationships. This is what that nurse caring for my mother in the intensive care unit acknowledged in her actions: my mother loved us, and we loved her. That nurse, that wonderful nurse, respected my mother's relationships. Even if a person is a recluse or is homeless, she or he still has relationships. After all, she or he has a relationship with you if you are her or his nurse. "To respect a person," Farley says, "is to respect her fundamental capacities for relationships as well as the relationships that are part of her concrete reality in the here and now." To be in the presence of the person who is our patient is to recognize her or his capacity for relationships and, as the nurse, to be in relationship with her or him.

This does not mean that we have to be emotionally involved. Indeed, being overinvolved emotionally can impede our ability to function as a nurse. Nor will we want to be friends with every person for whom we care; it is just a fact that we will not feel an affinity with every patient. We may lose patience with some patients. We may even find some patients repulsive: their views about society may not be ours; they may be so unkempt that their bodily odors make us gag. However, none of the difficulties of being in a relationship with a person as a nurse need get in the way of recognizing that we provide nursing care to people who, by virtue of being people, have the capacity to make decisions and to be in relationships.

We are people, too. We are vulnerable to disease and disorder, to natural disasters and accidents, and to the degradation of that which sustains our lives. Part of what makes the stranger-on-the-plane experience so powerful is that, in the moment of turbulence, we recognize that we share the same vulnerability as the person sitting next to us. I am a person, just as the stranger sitting next to me on the plane is a person. I am a person, just as the person in the hospital bed is a person. Not only are we vulnerable to disease and disorder but, just as with our patients, we have the capacities for self-determination and for relationships. We do not set these capacities aside when we become nurses. We are not just technically trained and board-certified nurses; we are people.

Nursing presence has been discussed in the nursing literature as an interpersonal process characterized by sensitivity, holism, intimacy, vulnerability, and uniqueness. To bring it about, the literature says, nurses must be willing and mature, must have moral underpinnings and a conducive work environment, and patients must be open and must need nursing presence. When it does occur, the literature says, it results in improved mental and physical well-being for those who experience it. I believe there is a phenomenon called "nursing presence," and I take the literature seriously about what it is. However, I seek to describe an experience that is both more primitive and more profound than the details of the literature suggest. The habit of presence is, amid all the busyness of the work of nursing, being a person with our patients, who, after all, are persons themselves.

PART II

THE ETHICAL
SIGNIFICANCE
OF NURSES' LIVES

The profession of nursing has a vision of a better world. In schools and clinics, in hospitals and homes, in community centers and colleges and universities, in the halls of policy-making institutions, and in makeshift highly infectious disease wards—we seek to bring this vision about through our acts of caring for and about people and their communities. What is good (acts of caring that bring about a better world) and what we ought to do (acts of caring that bring about a better world) become one in nursing. In this way, the "ought" (that which we ought to do in order to be good nurses) and the "is" (that which is good in and of itself) are the same in nursing. Because of this, ethics and nursing cannot be separated. Ethics is at the very core of nursing.

I have argued that we embody nursing's moral character by cultivating good habits in ourselves. I have investigated five such habits—trustworthiness, imagination, beauty, space, and presence. We seek to deliver competent, reliable, and honest nursing care, the components of the habit of trustworthiness. The habit of imagining a better world for our patients and their communities guides us on what care to offer. The habit of seeing our patients as beautiful drives us to bring justice to the injuries to their aliveness, even as they are dying; the habit of beauty shows that we care about—and for—the aliveness of our patients and their communities. We create the space in the place of care for patients to be as they are, instead of as defined by disease, disorder, disadvantage, or the dying process. Through the habit of presence, we see that we are not merely a health care professional working with someone who has a disease or a disorder or who is dying; we are a human being in the presence of another human being. Through the habit of presence, we share in our common humanity. The habits of trustworthiness, imagination, beauty, space, and presence embody nursing's moral character—caring about and for people and communities in order to bring about a better world for them.

So far I have explored the habits as we project them outward—toward patients' lives. But what difference do these five habits make in our own lives and among the community of nurses? In what follows, I explore how the habits of a good nurse can bring about a better world for us as a community of nurses. For I believe that the ethical significance of nursing rests not just in the profession's caring about and for patients and their communities but also in caring about and for the lives of our fellow nurses. It is to this we now turn—to the ethical significance of nurses' lives.

In Chapter 7, I speak about how the habit of trustworthiness helps us to meet the challenges of our work. In Chapter 8, we see how the habit of imagination can help us guard against the threat of becoming automated machines in the face of regimented technology. The harried and unrelenting nature of our work, its long shifts and emotional drain, can mean that we prefer others to ourselves; yet we matter, too. I suggest in Chapter 9 that the habit of seeing ourselves as beautiful is one way for us to bring justice to our own lives; we can be as good to ourselves as we are to our patients. In Chapter 10, we see that cultivating the habit of space creates a civil community of nurses. Finally, in Chapter 11, I suggest that practicing the habit of presence leads us to be grateful for the good—the good in the moment and the good we work to bring about.

We cultivate the habits of a good nurse not just to care for our patients but also to bring about nursing's ethos of caring among ourselves. In a profound way, the ethical significance of nurses' lives is that we cultivate the habits of a good nurse in ourselves in order to bring about a better nursing world. Habits are learned at the knee. Patricia Benner's novice-to-expert model is predicated upon the fundamental truth that expert nurses teach the habits of a good nurse to other nurses. That is, we pass on habits, and so, the habits we cultivate in ourselves will be the habits of the next generation of nurses. For the moral character of nursing to remain one invested in the primacy of caring about and for a better world for all, we have to live the habits of a good nurse within the community of nurses. In Chapter 12, I show that caring about and for a better world is the ethical significance of nurses' lives.

Chapter 7

The Challenge
of Unreasonable Demands

Two types of unreasonable demands confront us in our work as nurses. One demand is that of being a good nurse. Another is the work itself. Of course, they intertwine. For when we face unreasonable demands in our daily work, the demands of being a good nurse may become unreasonable, too. How can you, when you feel tired and grouchy, be good? How can you be a good nurse when you do not know the new electronic health record? How can you be a good nurse in the mind of the patient who yells at you for not coming to his or her room quick enough, especially when he or she calls for you three, four, or five times an hour? How can you be a good nurse when your nurse manager says you have to stay late to cover the shift of someone who did not show up? The demands of work may seem to make the demands of being good nearly impossible.

But it is more than that. Being good may place on us unreasonable demands. For example, the duty not to lie, some may say, is unreasonable. Is it better to tell your colleague that, in fact, you do not wish to help her or him turn the obese patient in room 2 just minutes before the end of your shift or to get your hands dirty with a lie, saying that you have to leave on time tonight because you have an appointment you cannot miss? You had already helped your colleague twice that day; your back is already on edge from heavy lifting; and your appointment is with the couch and a good television show. Is it not better to sully yourself with the lie? Your colleague would be hurt by the truth, you may say to yourself. Does not the lie serve a greater purpose than the truth? The contemporary philosopher Simon Blackburn cautions, however, that there is "something grubby . . . about the excuse that this argument gives." He comes down on the side of the truth, saying that "we should keep our own hands clean, however much others will dirty theirs." This is all well and good if we are talking about moral duties, such as the duty not to lie. But I am not talking about moral duties when I talk about habits. Habits suggest something other than duties.

The difference between a duty and a habit is that a duty is unbreakable, but a habit is an external sign of an inward devotion. Of course, there are times when circumstances get the best of us and we do not display the habits we have been trying to cultivate in ourselves, even though our devotion to nursing remains strong. We use these times as chances for growth.

Amelia, a certified oncology nurse I knew well, was working one day on an inpatient medical oncology floor. She began her shift one morning with four patients in four different rooms. Two patients were very sick; in fact, one of them was actively dying. The other two patients were in for rounds of chemotherapy. The dying patient's pain was not well managed, and the family kept pressing the call button, even though Amelia had told them that she had given their loved one all the pain medication that had been ordered. Amelia had paged the resident; she needed him to put in an order in the hospital's computerized charting system for an increased dose of the opiate the patient was on. It had been a good forty-five minutes without a reply; she had paged him twice, in fact, to no avail.

The other sick patient was admitted the previous night with a low white blood cell count, and Amelia needed to draw blood to send to the lab to see the patient's white blood cell count this morning. But first, it was critical that she get one of the other patients started on chemotherapy. The infusion took all day, and she needed to get it going so that it could be done before the night nurse came on. She wheeled in the standing scale, got the patient up out of bed, and weighed him. She wrote the weight down on the back of her hand. She used this weight and the height that was recorded in his chart, 188 centimeters, to calculate the patient's body surface area, from which the pharmacy would derive the exact dose of chemotherapy to administer. She had to calculate this using the calculator on her smartphone as the charting system, an older system, was not set up to handle such a calculation. It involved multiplying, dividing, and then taking a square root. As with protocol, another nurse had to double-check her calculations before she sent the patient's body surface area to the pharmacy. The calculations checked out, but the problem was that, in her busyness, Amelia had transposed numbers in the patient's weight. Instead of using 87 kilograms, his actual weight, she used 78 kilograms. Even though her calculations were correct, the result was wrong for this patient. The pharmacist who got Amelia's result for the patient's body surface area knew something was amiss. If she had used Amelia's result, the chemotherapy dose would have been much less than what she would have expected for this patient. The pharmacist called up to the floor and, instead of speaking directly to Amelia, spoke to the nurse manager. After hanging up the phone, the nurse manager called Amelia to the breakroom, and there, the manager lit into Amelia. How dare she be so incompetent! The patient could have gotten a wrong dose of chemotherapy, too low of a dose in this case, and thus an ineffective dose. "We are here to cure patients of their cancer, not give them a dose of chemo that won't do any good! You know, Amelia, I used to think I could trust you. I used to think you were a good nurse. But after today, I don't know." The nurse manager wrote an incident report. It was a five-copy form, white on top, then pink, yellow, light blue, and lastly, a gray copy that went in her file. Amelia read the report and signed it.

That day, as with so many days, Amelia's work demands were unreasonable. That she transposed a number in the craziness of that morning was understandable. Although understandable, it was still a mistake. Amelia wanted to give up right then and there. She wanted to walk off the job and go home. She felt embarrassed and, yes, incompetent. Yet she trudged through the day with an attention to detail the likes of which she had not had since she was a novice nurse; she was on her toes about every little thing. She also told the patient what had happened. She joked with him that she helped him lose 9 kilograms (about 20 pounds) in no time at all. But then, soberly and honestly, she explained everything she did. She explained how there were checks in their processes to make sure that he would get the right dose of chemotherapy. She apologized about it taking so long to get started and that he would probably still be getting his chemotherapy at bedtime, but at least it would be the right dose. The patient thanked her for her honesty and then told her not to worry about it anymore.

Unreasonable work demands lead to poorer patient outcomes. We know that higher nurse-to-patient ratios improve quality of care, including patient mortality in the hospital, even among the sickest of patients. We also know that hospital work environments in which nurses are recognized for good work and treated as peers with other health care professionals improve the quality of patient care. It is not that Amelia had proven herself untrustworthy but, rather, that the system had primed her to make a mistake that any human could make. She had too many very sick patients, and rather than treating her as a peer and going straight to her, the pharmacist went to her nurse manager, who seemed all too ready to assume the worst of Amelia.

Under the pressure of unreasonable demands, a trustworthy nurse can end up doing what Amelia did. A trustworthy nurse can make mistakes. However, when a nurse makes a mistake, a good nurse finds the habit of trustworthiness and wears it openly. Amelia was honest with the nurse manager and the patient; she admitted her mistake. She reliably went on with the rest of the day, with a hyper-acuity to the details of her work. To this day, Amelia checks and double-checks patients' weights and heights and her calculations; she is one of the most careful—and competent—nurses I know.

Making mistakes can lead to growth in competence, as it did with Amelia. Psychologists tell us that children who approach mistakes as opportunities for growth are more likely to succeed later in life. Scholars of technology tell us that failure is important to the process of innovation, if one looks at failure as a chance to go at the problem again until one finds a new method—or a solution to whatever one is working on. In health care, some mistakes lead to death. This is why we have safety checkpoints so that one person's mistake is not catastrophic. Amelia used her mistake to cultivate in herself competence, reliability, and honesty, the three components of trustworthiness we discussed in Chapter 2. The same could have been true of the nurse manager: how was this mistake a staffing failure? Amelia had one very sick and one dying patient. After all, these two patients alone could have kept Amelia busy the entire shift. How was Amelia's mistake also a failure of the system in which she was overburdened during this shift? In this situation, a root-cause analysis was indeed used to identify the systemic sources of failure, and the hospital took the right action, namely, putting flags in the electronic health record for a weight change greater than ten percent in any one-month period. From Amelia's mistake came necessary workplace innovations. The more we use mistakes and failures as opportunities to improve the workplace, the more we create the conditions necessary for nurses to be good.

Trustworthiness comes over time. Competence is not instantaneous. It takes education and years of gaining and proving nursing knowledge and clinical skills to become a competent nurse. It takes passing the nursing board. Then it takes training and proving skills-based competence on the floor. It takes showing up on time and practicing competently day after day. It takes doing what you say you will do—to your managers, to your colleagues, and to your patients. And it takes treating patients fairly. Trustworthiness is a process. Indeed, trustworthiness is a habit we put on over time. As with all habits, it is a set of behaviors to which we go when the system places unreasonable demands on us.

Trustworthiness is not just a personal habit. It is a habit of the community of nurses. When one of us does not know what to do, what to expect, or how to do something, we go to our nursing colleagues. "Have you ever seen a patient with this reaction from that medication?" we might ask another nurse. "Yes, I have," and on she or he goes to tell us about it. In this exchange, one nurse lifts the competence of another nurse. The competence of another lifts ours. "The competence of a group," the philosopher Torsten Wilholt writes, "can exceed the competence of even its most competent members." And so it is with reliability. One nurse may not show up for a shift, but the rest do and pitch in. One nurse might be too busy, say, with a very sick patient who has a lot going on, to answer the call of another patient, but she or he reaches out to a colleague who has a moment to stick her or his head into the patient's room. "Your nurse is busy with another patient right now. How may I help you?" We have all done that for each other. The same is true for reliability. When one nurse proves unreliable, we step in to show patients our reliability as a community of nurses. The same is true with honesty. Indeed, the work of nursing is predicated on honesty. In instances in which one nurse might seek to deceive, we take action as a group. We do not abide deception in the community of nurses, for we know that we cannot be nurses and be dishonest. In those times in which it is very difficult to be honest with patients, as it was for Amelia to be honest with her patient about why it took so long to get his chemotherapy started, the community supports us. I remember when I was a novice nurse practitioner and was about do a procedure alone for the first time, my mentor told me to be honest with the patient. "Tell him this is your first time to do it unaided. Tell him that I'll be standing right there, in case you need help." Deep down, I was afraid to tell my patient; I did not want to look green, but more so, I did not want to admit my fear. With my mentor's prodding, however, I was honest with my patient, and he was magnanimous, which, I have learned time and time again, most patients are. My mentor nurse practitioner emboldened me to be honest. We, the community of nurses, help each other to be more competent, more reliable, and more honest nurses. In the community of nurses, we find the strength to be trustworthy nurses—more strength than we often have alone.

As a community we have gone to the habit of trustworthiness in the most difficult of situations. The nurses in West Africa who showed up to work during the Ebola crisis, who risked their own lives to care for the lives of others, are paragons of trustworthiness. Even though we can speak about individual nurses who provided trustworthy nursing care in that devastating health crisis, we speak about the collective, the group. That group of Ebola nurses was trustworthy. "The trustworthiness of the group," Wilholt says, "cannot be reduced to the trustworthiness of its members." The trustworthiness of one nurse does not make all nurses trustworthy, but rather, the trustworthiness of the community of nurses is more than the trustworthiness of just one of us alone. This is the power of the profession of nurses.

We are trustworthy as nurses because patients need us to be trustworthy. Their care—and their health—depends on our competence, our reliability, and our honesty. Yet there is something more profound about the trustworthiness of nurses. We call society to trustworthiness. Health is necessary for the good society. Yet too often the conditions people live in do not promote health. We, the largest of the health professions, can stand up for health care policy that promotes health. Public officials must ensure that drinking water is not tainted with lead or other chemicals that damage health. Public officials must ensure that food is safe and that people have access to quality food—to fresh fruit and vegetables. People who live in areas that do not have grocery stores or farmers' markets that sell fresh produce, so-called food deserts, have higher obesity rates. Moreover, people who live in food deserts tend to be people of color. Nurses need to address these and other issues of health care policy, with the same trustworthiness they address individual patient care. The trustworthiness of nursing is founded upon our being trustworthy for all people, regardless of who they are or where they live. The profession of nursing, by having a vision of the good society of better health for all people and by working to that end, offers a vision of a trustworthy society, especially for those for whom society has not historically proven itself trustworthy.

In the Ebola ward, in the refugee camp, at the disaster scene, in the halls of power, or in the clinic, nurses deal with unreasonable demands. The system, insofar as it is a system, will at times burden us with unreasonable demands. Patients, insofar as they are vulnerable and need our care, will at times place unreasonable demands upon us. At times, our home lives will also place unreasonable demands on us. Yet the community of nurses is the well from which we can draw the sustenance to carry on as trustworthy nurses, for each other, for our patients, and for society.

We as a nursing community face another challenge. In an age of automated treatment algorithms and flags on the electronic health record, which can prevent errors—as we saw with Amelia—we face the threat of becoming a mere extension of this automation, losing our own ability to make clinical decisions. As we find out in the next chapter, however, the habit of imagination protects against this threat. We use our imaginations to establish for ourselves and for our patients and their communities an image of health restored or promoted or an image of safely passing from this life. Imagination can never be automated. Imagination keeps our nursing care human.

The Threat of Becoming Automatons

We have the ability to make clinical decisions. That is why we went to nursing school, after all, to use our brains to make decisions about the care of people. However, once we registered as a nurse, we took on more than this ability; we took on clinical responsibility. We often feel the weight of this responsibility, especially the more we have to worry about details such as charting, making patients happy, and knowing how to apply the latest evidence. One way we are tempted to deal with the weight of this responsibility is to do exactly what we are told. Sometimes, we do just what the questions on the electronic chart tell us in order to make sure we do what is required of us, not necessarily what makes for good care. We do what we must for our patients to give us good marks on the patient satisfaction survey—without thinking about what is best to do in the situation. And we follow care algorithms to a tee—even if deviating makes sense for some patients. We fear messing up. It is a real fear; I feel it, too. But when we respond to this fear by following electronically generated assessment questions and scripts and algorithms without using our own brains in specific clinical situations, we risk becoming automatons. The irony is, if we let ourselves become automatons in an attempt not to mess up under the weight of our responsibilities, we end up surrendering the very responsibility that makes us nurses. Let me explain.

Amelia, the oncology nurse we met in Chapter 6 who transposed numbers in a patient's weight, needed the benefits of electronic charting. Indeed, electronic charting's flags about sudden weight change now serve as a safety check, and its ability to do complex medical math equates with fewer calculation errors. At the same time, electronic charting makes sure that nurses are thorough in their assessments. But these benefits of electronic charting, particularly routine assessment questions, can take the human element out of a nurse's care.

It used to be that pain was not routinely assessed. Some patients suffered in silence. But then pain was understood to be the fifth vital sign, and nurses had to assess for pain every time they took patients' blood pressure, heart and respiration rates, and temperature. Amelia now feels that automatic assessment questions, though meant to make sure she is thorough, potentially take away from her hands-on assessment.

In the old days, Amelia would assess her patients while providing hands-on care. She would assess for the presence of pain, its level on the numeric pain scale, its physical location, and its quality while giving a bed bath. "What does the pain here feel like?" She could ask when the pain began; whether it waxed or waned; whether it radiated to other parts of the body; what other symptoms went with it, especially emotional symptoms such as depression and anxiety; and what, if anything, made it worse or better. We know these as the seven dimensions that characterize a symptom: its chronology, bodily location, quality, quantity, setting, associated manifestations, and aggravating or alleviating factors. These seven dimensions help us to gain a clearer picture of what is going on with patients who tell us they are in pain. Asking these questions takes clinical acumen.

A nurse moves between the dimensions during her assessment, putting disparate information together to arrive at a clearer clinical picture.

Now, in the days of electronic charting, Amelia wheels the computer into the patient's room and follows the questions on the screen. She asks the patient "the pain question"—"Please rate your pain on a scale of zero to ten"—while looking at the computer screen so that she can make sure the cursor is in the right place. Then she clicks on the box with the number that accords with the patient's answer. She waits a few seconds for the hourglass to go away, indicating that the entry has uploaded in the patient's electronic chart somewhere on "the cloud." She goes to the next question, and again, she looks at the computer screen as she clicks on the box that matches the patient's answer and waits for the entry to upload. These electronic questions standardize nursing assessment. There is comfort in the certitude of a standardized assessment. However, we can let this certitude turn our assessment into an automatic activity, instead of a patient-care activity.

The assessment questions of electronic charting are helpful. In the busyness of the hospital and the clinic, they ensure that we do not forget important aspects of clinical care, such as assessing patients for pain. The issue is whether we let assessment questions, instead of nurses, become the interface with patients. We can let questions turn us into automated nurses who conduct automatic assessments. We can do just what they tell us to do—and nothing more. That is, we can let electronic charting automate our interactions with patients. We can surrender our human responsibility to the machine and become automatons. In that way, we can surrender our clinical responsibility of care.

The word "clinical" can conjure up cold, unemotional, and detached treatment. If we relinquish our clinical responsibility to the logic and the prompts of the chart, our work does become detached. However, the word "clinical" also means the actual care of people in the setting of the hospital, the clinic, the school, the home. We can use the electronic chart as a guide for our care of people as they seek health or a peaceful death. We can use it to make sure we do not forget to assess for pain but still assess for pain in the hands-on way that we know is good clinical care. We can view the logic and the prompts of the electronic chart as signposts on the path of nursing imagination we talked about in Chapter 3, the kind of imagination in which we feel what the patient feels. When we provide human-oriented care while using the modern technology of automatic assessment questions, it is as if we say to ourselves, "I am asking the patient about pain, but let me imagine what she or he feels and how I may go about ameliorating her or his pain." This approach establishes sympathy with the patient; it establishes the common feeling of our humanity. When we use the automation of the electronic chart in this way, we are not an automaton doing just what the prompts of the electronic chart require; we are humans caring for humans.

The demands of charting are indeed great. Charting does take an enormous amount of our time, and we must be careful in our charting. But charting cannot take the place of providing human care.

As with charting, so with our concerns about patient satisfaction. The concern to make sure patients give us, our hospitals, and our clinics high ratings on patient satisfaction surveys can, if we let it, drive us into becoming automatons. Popular health care writer Alexandra Robbins highlights this concern in her essay "The Problem with Satisfied Patients." Some payers are now basing reimbursements to hospitals on patient satisfaction. Surveys that assess patient satisfaction largely focus on the care that we nurses deliver. One risk, Robbins points out, is that patients become customers, demanding what they want. What they want may not always be good nursing care, based upon the whole clinical situation. Patients do not always have the knowledge and skills to determine whether what they want in the moment accords with their goals of care in the long term or is at cross purposes with their health. An example Robbins gives is of a patient who had just had coronary bypass surgery complaining to his nurse that he did not get enough pastrami on his sandwich. The exchange between the I-want-more-pastrami patient and his nurse escalated, Robbins reports, and the patient became dissatisfied.

We can be tempted, in times such as these, to give in to patients' demands for the sake of higher patient satisfaction scores. Yet the intent of patient satisfaction is not that patients subvert the process of providing sound nursing care; it is, rather, to empower and activate patients to take charge of their care. This view of patient care emancipates patients from a paternalistic approach—"You must not eat pastrami!"—to a dialogue-centered approach. Why did the patient consent to heart surgery? Surely this included the goal of a longer, healthier life. Then can we work with the patient to agree upon what she or he needs to do in order to achieve his goal of a longer, healthier life? This can be difficult; some patients just want more pastrami regardless of why they came into the hospital. But ultimately it is not about pastrami; it is about empowering and activating the patient to become a better steward of her or his health. It is tempting to be driven by the patient satisfaction survey and give in to what the patient wants, but if we do that, we become automatons of the patient satisfaction survey. If what patients want does not agree with why patients are in the hospital or clinic, then we can aim to provide the kind of care that empowers and activates patients to do what accords with their goals of care.

Remember how the habit of imagination we discussed in Chapter 3 is intrinsic to Virginia Henderson's concept of nursing?

We have to imagine what patients would do for themselves if they had the will, knowledge, or power to restore or promote their health. If they do not have the knowledge, then good nursing care educates them about how to promote or restore their health. If they do not have the will, then good nursing care provides them a sense of agency for health. If they do not have the strength, then good nursing care builds them up. Nursing imagination can use the moments in which patients could tip over into dissatisfaction for moral imagination, empowering and activating patients to take charge of their health promotion or restoration.

It is not just charting and the push for greater patient satisfaction survey scores that can, if we practice without nursing imagination, trap us into practicing nursing as automatons. Evidence-based practice guidelines can, too. Such guidelines are determined through systematic reviews and meta-analyses in which randomized controlled trials are given the heaviest weight. A randomized controlled trial tells us whether an intervention produces better results in patients who receive it than in patients who do not receive it. It is important to practice in accordance with the evidence, as discovered in rigorous randomized controlled trials. Yet such trials are, as their name suggests, well controlled. Patients' lives are not so well controlled. For instance, some patients' bodies may react strongly to a novel medical treatment that trials have found works for different conditions, and sometimes, some of the patients who receive a new medical treatment do not get the same results as the patients who were studied in the trials. Studies of randomized controlled trials report aggregated results. However, an individual patient is not an aggregate.

I had a patient who had an aggressive form of cancer for which there was a new treatment that in a trial extended survival by a little over two weeks. The medical team presented the evidence to the patient and offered the treatment as the next step in care. When

I spoke with the patient, she told me that she was too tired. She did not want the treatment. She was ready to switch her care from anti-cancer care to end-of-life care. In my role as the nurse practitioner, I served as the intermediary between the medical team and the patient. The medical team had a difficult time understanding her decision. They had good evidence that the treatment extended life. However, the evidence that the team offered her was not evidence for her. She had a life-limiting disease. Her life was short; this she knew. She was ready to die. Two weeks more of life, even if it was a good two weeks, were not worth it for her.

Evidence-based guidelines that are derived from rigorous and important trials may not be evidence for everyone. We often cannot see this unless we imagine what it is like for the patient. My patient had been a triathlete. She had run marathons, swum miles, and biked even farther. Living two more weeks—even a full twelve more months—in her condition was not worth it for her. To understand her I had to imagine the joy she found from moving her body. Her children were grown. She had lived her life, and living it to her meant moving her body, which she could no longer do. I had had patients for whom two more weeks of life would have meant everything. They would have gone for the treatment. But not this particular patient. To understand that, I had to imagine her suffering from not being able to move her body, a condition we would not improve with the novel medication. We have to imagine the lives of our patients to understand just when evidence is not evidence for them, and then, we must implement the evidence in a way that makes sense in the context of their lives. We treat patients, not statistical results. We can imagine the lives of patients, not frequencies, percentages, means, and Kaplan-Meier curves. This we must keep in mind in order not to practice as automatons.

There are, however, public health considerations in which evidence is evidence for everyone. Vaccines against communicable diseases are good for all. People who do not get vaccinated put in peril others around them whose health, perhaps because of an immunocompromised state, would worsen or life be threatened, should they contract such diseases. It is as much a failure of imagination to think that not vaccinating oneself or one's child against publicly spread diseases will have no consequence for others.

However, in the cases in which evidence is not evidence for everyone, practicing as though it were strips us of the human aspects of nursing, the imaginative aspects of our practice. It is a failure of imagination when we let the logic of electronic charting, the drive for patient satisfaction survey results, and evidence-based algorithms drive our practice. The well-designed and carefully run randomized controlled trial is important; it determines whether an intervention is more effective than the way we normally practice. It is also important that patients are satisfied with the care they receive. On the one hand, this may mean that they did not have to wait too long for clinical appointments; but on the other, it may mean that we have helped them to see that the care we give them will promote or restore their health, even if the result is not immediately apparent. In addition, the logical consistency and the standardized assessment questions of electronic charting serve as a safety checklist. My concern, however, is that, amid these important advances, the humanity of nursing must not be lost, the humanity of understanding the significance of another person's sufferings—of understanding the significance of another person's journey through this life.

This is the power of our lives as nurses: we can imagine the lives of our patients. For it is in imagining their lives—their hopes and their joys, their sorrows and their sufferings—that we become nurses in the fullest sense. Balanced against this is our real fear of uncertainty in our daily lives as nurses. We can seek certitude as an antidote to our fears, but certainty born of fear is false. Following standardized assessment questions exactly, without doing a more in-depth assessment, lures us into the false certainty of doing what we are supposed to do. Getting more pastrami for the patient, even if it is not good for his health, may not result in a patient who rates us poorly on the patient satisfaction survey; but it also may not result in a patient with restored health. Following the evidence-based algorithm that suggests offering a certain medical treatment may calm our fears of not practicing according to the science, but it may not be science that makes sense in the context of a patient's life. When we flee to certainty out of fear, we force all clinical situations into the same algorithms, even though they may not all fit. Certainty born of fear is the enemy of imagination. We need bravely to free our imaginations to understand our patients' lives and how our nursing care can promote or restore their health or lead them to a serene passing. When we practice with imagination we keep technology from becoming the tyrant that strips us of our humanity; imagination keeps technology in its place.

Nursing imagination establishes the hope of health promoted, health restored, or life safely passing. When we are able to help our patients achieve that, through our imagination, we have resisted the threat of becoming an automaton. This is the ethical significance of imagination in our everyday lives as nurses.

Through the habit of imagination, we preserve our patients' humanity in the world of automation and technology. We preserve our own as well. But to be human is to have doubts and fears; it is, at times, to make mistakes. Being human means we are vulnerable to injuries ourselves. As with our patients and their communities, however, beauty demands justice when it is injured. If not being an automaton means that we are vulnerable to injury, then our beauty as human beings stands there waiting for us to recognize that, though we can be injured, we, too, share in the rights of justice. Automation may be clean. It may be efficient and save costs. But it lacks beauty, in that it cannot lay claim to justice. We, as nurses who are fully human, are vulnerable to injury. We lay claim to justice by seeing the beauty of our humanity. In the next chapter, we discuss how we can do this.

Chapter 9

Being Good to Ourselves

When I have a hard day at work and I share my difficulties with colleagues, invariably one of them will tell me to be good to myself. When I hear this, I often picture a white sandy beach and an azure sea lapping the shore directly in front of a chaise lounge I find myself reclining on in the warm sun. As wonderful as this fantasy is, it is not what my colleagues mean when they tell me to be good to myself.

It can be difficult to be good to ourselves. A beach vacation may give us rest and take our minds off work for a week or two. A good foot massage will offer rest and relaxation, until the next twelve-hour shift. We can—and should—eat well and exercise, and we can take refuge in hobbies or in the confidence of good friends. All these are good and important strategies for self-care, which is part of what my colleagues mean when they tell me to be good to myself. However, it is not all of what they mean when they tell me this, for at the end of the day, there is no actual single thing we can do that will undo the myriad difficulties we face as nurses. A vacation, a spa experience, a good book, or collapsing in the arms of our loved ones do not prevent our patients from dying, being diagnosed with life-limiting disease, showing up in our emergency room having just been raped, or having births go wrong. Nor does self-care alone undo the exhaustion we face from our hard work. What my colleagues mean when they encourage me to be good to myself is, quite literally, to be ethical toward myself. They mean that I should recharacterize my life as a nurse in such a way that brings justice to the difficulties I experience on the job.

The power of stories in making sense of difficulties hit me most when my son was a little boy. When he had encountered difficulties during the day, he would often lie awake at night and dwell upon them. On these nights, he sometimes would ask me to come into his room, sit on the side of his bed, and tell him a story about when something similar had happened to me. Typically, before I was finished telling my story, he would drift off to sleep. Either my voice was soporific or he was reassured that he would be all right, just as I was all right in the story I told him about myself. Of course, with my long view, I had faith that he would make it through the difficulty at hand. But eventually I came to realize that something more was going on in my telling the stories of my surviving my childhood difficulties: I benefited from telling these stories as much as my son did, perhaps even more. Of course, I remembered the injuries of my childhood—the embarrassing moments, the painful moments, the moments I encountered bullies on the playground, the moments of betrayal by people I thought were my friends. I began the stories with these injuries, but somehow, unconsciously, I ended the stories with justice. Sometimes I ended them with the justice brought about by others on my behalf, sometimes by how I overcame my injuries by tenacity and hard work and, when my injuries were at the hand of another person, by forgiveness. Even when the injuries were at my own hand (my dog, after all, did not eat the homework I forgot to do), I ended the story by forgiveness. Eventually, I came to see that telling our stories reminds us that when we are injured, justice heals.

We may experience injury when people place unjust demands on us. I was a new nurse working on a team in which the physician on fellowship (also known as the "fellow") on the team had a lot of latitude to tell others what to do. A patient needed to have a peripherally inserted central catheter (PICC line) removed. Even though it was a simple procedure, the hospital required nurses to be trained and certified in the procedure before performing it. I was not. The trained and certified nurse was busy; she would not be able to remove the patient's PICC line for about an hour. The patient would have to wait. The fellow grew irritated at me and, in front of the patient, "ordered" me to do it. I refused, giving my reason of not being certified. There were possible complications, some life-threatening, if the line was not removed according to procedure. My refusal strained my relationship with the fellow, and for the next several months, he treated me unkindly.

At first, it was hard for me to find justice in the story. The fellow had made my clinical life difficult. However, after telling this story over and over to my colleagues, I realized that it was justice that, when she arrived, the trained and certified nurse who took out the patient's PICC line defended my refusal to do so to the patient. It was justice that the patient was not subjected to undue risk of complication. After the tensions between the fellow and me did not abate over the several intervening months, my nurse manager confronted him about his behavior; this, too, was justice. Later, as the patient was preparing to leave the care of the team and proceed to hospice for end-of-life care, the patient and I had an exchange in which he thanked me for the care I had given him. The patient himself said that he was glad I had said no to the fellow. The patient gave me a gift when he told me this; it was, perhaps, the greatest justice for the injury of being ordered to perform unsafe practice. As I tell this story now, I am healed anew by the justice with which others salved my injury, especially the patient; they saw me as beautiful, a person who, by virtue of my humanity, is worthy of justice. But more so, I am healed by the fact that the injustice was not allowed to injure the beauty of the patient.

The more I retell this and other nursing stories, the more I understand the meaning of justice in my nursing practice. Justice is that which is right, both in the sense of the right way to practice and in the sense of righting wrongs, that is, making injustices right. In the situation with the fellow, I had practiced rightly by not removing the PICC line, and my community of nurses had set right the wrong of the fellow's behavior. Justice is also fairness. It was fair to the patient that I did not perform a procedure I was not trained and certified to do. It was also fair to myself, for had I performed the procedure, I would have put myself in jeopardy. Justice is that which is right and fair, and that which is right and fair is beautiful. Justice not only restores beauty when it has been injured, acts of restoring rightness and fairness to someone are good acts, acts that restore beauty. There was goodness in the acts of the people involved in this situation, which I only uncovered by telling and retelling the story, a story that began with an injury that was painful for me for a long time but ended with rightness and fairness, that is, with beauty being restored. We are good to ourselves when, in telling the stories of injuries committed against us, we search for and find justice, for justice restores beauty.

I have over the years tried to understand the fellow's actions. Perhaps his actions were motivated by wanting the best for his patient, insofar as he did not want his patient to wait. Perhaps he felt insecure: as a fellow, he was in training, and he should have had more oversight by the attending (also known as "consulting") physicians who were training him. Maybe the fellow was stressed from other issues going on in the clinic and lost control of himself. Maybe the fellow just acted badly. Without any check, we can surprise even ourselves, at times, by the impulse within us to behave badly; it seemingly comes out of nowhere, and without tamping it down, we can unthinkingly act on it. We must check our primitive urges. This check does not have to be external, though the attending physicians who supervised the fellow could have provided an external check for him. However, the fellow could have provided this check for himself; indeed, most often impulse control needs to come from within ourselves.

The cousin of the primitive urge to behave savagely is the primitive urge to study human evil, that is, to try to understand people's acting on their primitive urges for savage behavior. I spent a good deal of my life as a philosopher studying the problem of evil, and I have no answer. But I have come to believe that we all have within us an urge to act savagely; we all have the ability to commit injurious acts. However, the urge to study human evil serves the purpose of keeping ourselves from acting on these savage impulses. And here we see one reason we should tell the stories of the injurious things other people do to us: in telling these stories, we ponder why people commit injurious deeds in order to check ourselves. These stories of injuries become, for us and for those to whom we tell them, a lesson in how not to act. This is the importance of not forgetting even the most unfathomable and horrible events. We must remember these horrible events, for in remembering we provide a check. Telling these stories saves ourselves from our baser natures and makes us better people. There is a paradox here: when we tell the stories of the injuries of our lives, we are being good to ourselves; for by telling stories of immoral behavior, we subdue the savagery in ourselves.

We tell stories from our point of view. The other characters in our stories, though real, do not have a say in how we tell our stories. Without their side of the story, our versions can end up demonizing others. Our stories can devolve into war stories. This is not the purpose of telling the stories of the difficulties we face in our work as nurses. Rather, if we are to choose beauty over injury, justice over injustice, we should take care to tell our stories in ways that remind ourselves that we all face difficulties. The fellow I worked with, to be sure, faced difficulties. Telling the story of our interaction, however, reminds us—me, him, and you—that there is a just (indeed, a trustworthy) way to act. Telling stories of injustice offers us the chance to imagine that which is just. In this way, I believe that justice triumphs over savagery. Some savagery is too great for any undoing of it, particularly wanton taking of life. However, I believe that we must remember even the most injurious of stories and use them to guide our behavior.

It is not only others who can act unjustly toward us; we can also act unjustly toward ourselves. A friend of mine, a critical care nurse, told me a story of a young adult patient of hers who had been admitted for an as yet unspecified cardiac arrhythmia. The nurse told me that she was certain the cardiac care team would identify the problem and fix it; she was certain her patient would recover. The nurse imagined her patient leaving the intensive care unit, going home, and living the rest of her life in health. However, the patient went into cardiac arrest, and although the team tried to resuscitate her, it could not. My friend told and retold this story to me, asking the rhetorical question of what she had done wrong. She replayed the scene over and over. "What did I miss? What clinical sign did I not see?" Then my friend passed judgment on herself: "I should have seen it coming. If only I had done this or that." My friend walked around with her judgment of how she did not save her patient. My friend judged herself unjustly, yet she had provided good nursing care, the care any reasonable nurse would provide. The problem with judging ourselves unjustly is that, when we do, we injure ourselves. When we injure ourselves, we cannot find the beauty in the care we have provided.

Search for one moment when your nursing care promoted or restored a person's health or afforded safe passage from this life. Take time to recall it in as much detail as possible. Let it fill your mind. Find the beauty in this moment. Now find other moments like it. These moments come together to form a beautiful picture of your work as a nurse. Finding the beauty in your work as a nurse saves you from treating yourself unjustly, for beauty, as Augustine said, saves us on life's rough seas. Beauty breaks the frame of our unjust judgments against ourselves. A young woman dying is unjust, under any circumstances; and when this happens on our shift, we feel its weight. However, remembering beautiful moments of providing trustworthy nursing care to her lifts the weight. When something goes wrong and you, though not at fault, unjustly judge yourself, you can be good to yourself by remembering the moments that you provided good nursing care.

Other people injure us, and we injure ourselves. But there are times when we could have acted differently. We lash out at well-meaning colleagues in the heat of the moment. We do miss clinical signs. We do make mistakes. We are, after all, human. In these situations, we must own up to our mistakes. The nursing profession has well-developed processes to identify the causes of mistakes and change policies and procedures so that the same mistakes do not occur again. We admit our mistakes so that these processes can take effect, for the sake of our patients' and our own safety. In this way, admitting our mistakes is a way of being good to ourselves and to others. Admitting our mistakes is part of what it means to be a trustworthy nurse, for a trustworthy nurse is honest and imagines herself or himself learning from mistakes.

There are indeed times in which the profession has to say that a nurse's practice is so unsafe that she or he cannot continue to practice. Few worse fates can befall a nurse, for, as I have argued, nursing becomes who we are; it becomes our identity. Being stripped of the ability to work as a nurse is to be stripped of a part of one's self. But when this must be the case, the person can be good to herself or himself by no longer practicing as a nurse, for who wants one's practice to result in grievous injury to colleagues or to patients, or even worse, to be the cause of a patient's demise?

When injustices are committed against us or when we commit injustices against ourselves, we are good to ourselves when we tell our stories and find justice and beauty in our work as nurses. We are good to ourselves when we admit mistakes and when we realize the limits of our safety. However, we are also good to ourselves when we ponder the good of our nursing care. Let me explain.

When I told my son the stories of my childhood, stories that had to do with universal experiences of figuring out how we live in the world, which can, at times, be truculent, I always ended the stories with how justice healed my injuries. These were not fairy tales or fantasies. I was sitting on his bed, after all, having survived the injuries the stories were about. Sometimes, when I conjured up the injuries of my childhood, decades later, the pain still felt deep. But with each story, greater than the pain was the awe I felt at the fact that my story always ended in the present with my son and me in his room. That fact was—and still is—proof enough that justice heals. It was always a beautiful moment, a moment of healing. By the time the story ended, my son had nodded off to sleep, and I walked out of his bedroom a grown man who had survived the injuries of childhood. I was awestruck each time. The same is true with the beautiful moments of our nursing care: they heal our injuries. And they strike awe in us—awe at there being good in what we do, awe in the good of our simple acts of nursing care. Being awestruck at how good—how ethical—our daily work as nurses is, is another way we can be good to ourselves.

Awe is difficult to describe. It is respect, but it is also surprise mixed with an awareness of our place in the world. The starry sky above inspired awe in Immanuel Kant, the philosopher whose association of awe with morality I mentioned in Chapter 4. I grew up on the desert. On dark, clear nights, I loved to stand alone on the desert sands and look up at the sky. Some nights, I could see the Milky Way, the spiraled galaxy that contains our solar system. It was a breathtaking sight. I would feel small, not small in the sense of insignificant but small in the sense of standing in the presence of something so vast. I would feel my place in the grand scheme of things. Without anyone telling me, I knew this feeling. It was awe, awe at there being what there is, and awe that I am a part of it.

Not only did the starry sky above inspire awe in Kant, but so did what he called the moral law within. We do not need to go into what Kant meant by this to agree with him that when we experience good, we feel awe. Beauty, awe, and good are bound up together. Think of the justice you bring to the lives of people who have been touched with disease and disorder; that is, think of how your nursing care restores beauty to them. This is good, in the moral sense. Now when you see this good, be filled with awe—awe at there being good in what you do, awe at the cumulative effects of the good of nursing around the world. The good that comes from nurses everywhere forms a galaxy of goodness. Find your place in that galaxy of goodness. Feel awe at being a part of it.

Nursing involves mundane tasks. It also involves wonderful moments, moments of birth and aliveness. But it involves injury, too. Justice and beauty and goodness and awe are powerful friends against the daily grit of nursing. Be good to yourself by finding these powerful friends in your stories as a nurse. The more I reflect upon my nursing stories, the more I am awestruck at the beauty, justice, and good my nursing practice results in. The same can be true for you. Reflect upon your work as a nurse and the good that comes from it. Tell your nursing stories over and over, until you can feel awe at what you do. This is yet another way to be good—that is ethical—toward yourself: tell your nursing stories and feel awe at the good that you do.

Chapter 10

Creating a Civil Community

Heavy patient workloads, high patient acuity, and mountains of paperwork overwhelm us. Twelve-hour workdays, three in a row, leave little time at the end of the night to put our sore and achy feet up. We work in places in which there is a pecking order, and in some cases, we may have much more experience and real-life clinical knowledge than clinicians who rank higher in that pecking order. In teaching hospitals, negotiating with interns and residents can be tricky. Our patients are sicker than they have ever been; patient acuity has risen steadily, and hospital length-of-stay has fallen sharply. We have to get patients well enough to be discharged; that is our job. On top of all this, there is the phrase I am scared to write, but if I do not, I will be dishonest. We all know the phrase. If there were a book of common nursing adages, it would be the entry listed among the most commonly used: "Nurses eat their young." Yes, nurses can be bullies. Up to seventy percent of new nurses have reported experiencing uncivil behavior, and up to ninety percent of all nurses have reported experiencing uncivil behavior from other nurses.

The sources of stress in our jobs are many, and we can do something about them. There have been novel proposals about how to address workplace bullying, such as using low reimbursement rates to penalize institutions when nurses who work there report high levels of bullying. However, the issue of workplace bullying points to a larger concern, the concern of how we come together as a community of nurses.

The good society that Annie Goodrich envisioned was one in which the conditions for disease and disorder—such as poor sanitation, cramped living conditions, unsafe food and water, poverty, lack of education, and disrespect—were addressed by public service institutions, including, but especially for Goodrich, nursing. In Goodrich's view, the ultimate aim of nursing was to work to achieve the good society. Yet too often we find ourselves working in environments in which the very notion of the good society, a society in which people respect each other, is hard to come by. How can we, within our own community, live the good society we hope to bring about?

There is a straightforward answer to that question. The habit of creating a space for our patients to inhabit in the place of care is the same habit we cultivate in ourselves for each other as nurses. We create a space for each other, regardless of our individual particularities. This space is the community of nurses. One way we create this space is through civility.

The English word "civility" originates from the Latin word *civis*. *Civis* is also the root for the English word "citizen." Civility and citizenship, that is, share a parent; they carry the same word DNA. Let me explain their family resemblance. We treat other people with civility because we believe they have something about them that makes them worthy of treating them that way. That is, we treat other people with civility because they have what the contemporary philosopher Cheshire Calhoun calls a "morally considerable fact." Simply put, being human is a morally considerable fact, for being human comes with moral rights (about how one ought to be treated) and duties (about how one ought to treat others). The whole of humanity shares in these moral rights and duties. We all are citizens of the human community, and as such, we all have the right to be treated with civility. Moreover, we have the duty to treat others with civility. We treat people with civility because people are citizens of the human community.

We could say that we treat other nurses with civility because we are all nurses. However, our being nurses alone does not constitute a morally considerable fact that outweighs other qualities we have. It does indeed seem invidious and shocking that up to ninety percent of all nurses and seventy percent of new nurses have been treated uncivilly—by other nurses. Given these percentages, it must be that we behave uncivilly, even though we have been the recipient of other nurses' uncivil behavior toward us. The morally considerable fact that demands our treating other nurses with civility is not their status as nurses but, rather, their humanity. We all are citizens of the human community before we are citizens of the nursing community. When we are in the presence of other nurses, we are in the presence of other humans, humans who have the moral right to be treated with civility, humans who have the moral duty to treat others with civility. Civility displays our moral attitude of respect for humanity.

Civility is the outward sign of an inward respect for others. The civil nurse respects other nurses, regardless of their gender, their age, their skin color or ethnicity, their height or weight, their religion, their being a new grad or a nurse who has practiced for fifty years. We show this respect in two ways.

First, we refrain from uncivil behaviors. Such behaviors include rude and abusive language, gossiping and rumors, and discourteous behaviors such as refusing to help a colleague. Civility is also, at times, restraining speech. Our workplace is highly charged. One mistake and a patient might die. In one instance in which I was treated uncivilly, another nurse thought I was close to making a mistake. Yet the other nurse rebuked me with hostility, using foul language and name-calling. I experienced her rebuke as violating, for she lacked respect for me. In the breakroom after the incident, the other nurse spread around her opinion of me. She quite literally called me names in front of the other nurses in the breakroom, and then after the fact, she continued to talk poorly about me among others. To show respect is not to make comments about another nurse but, rather, to talk about the work of nursing. When they may make (or do make) a mistake, show respect by telling them why you think their action is a mistake. Civility, to the twentieth-century American philosopher John Rawls, requires that, when we disagree and overrule others, we explain why. Civility is to respect other nurses enough to explain your disagreement, to have an open conversation about nursing care.

However, civility does not have to equate with likability. As when we feel compassion toward our patients whether we like them or not—as described in Chapter 4—we do not have to enjoy the company of all nurses we work with or be friends with them. Indeed, we may find some people boring, or we may not have anything in common with them, other than being a nurse. But civil people do not convey these sentiments because civil people take others' feelings into account. Others may have different, though no less reasonable, ways of living and expressing themselves.

The second way to show respect is to listen to other nurses, to try to see things from their point of view. Perhaps a nurse was not about to make a mistake; perhaps she or he knew of new evidence supporting a different way of intervening in whatever was going on with the patient. Perhaps a nurse was indeed about to make a grave mistake but because of the hostile work environment, she or he was too afraid to ask what to do. To show civility in the community of nurses is to make it possible for nurses to talk and to listen without fear of reprisal. Indeed, there are times when we have to communicate why we think another nurse is about to make a mistake. Although we may do this as kindly as possible, the nurse may feel awful about it rather than feel good that she or he was spared a mistake or that we support her or him in learning from a mistake she did make. We do not need to turn a blind eye to impending or real mistakes out of fear of hurting another's feelings. It is, rather, out of respect for our fellow nurses that we help them. Civility requires that we help each other in such a way that we can learn and improve; it communicates to others our moral attitude that they are worthy of our interventions into their practice and, conversely, also means having the respect to listen to others and to communicate openly about our nursing practice without judgments.

It is not civil to hold stereotypes based on sex, gender, age, race, or other divisors we use to separate us from our common humanity. We call these divisors into question, for following them often results in uncivil behavior. A friend of mine went to nursing school the same time I did. He, like me, had had children already. He was well aware of childbirth and of what was involved after childbirth, particularly with breastfeeding. For his maternal–newborn clinical rotation, he was placed in a large academic hospital, along with four female nursing students from his school. None of these women had had previous experience with childbirth or with breastfeeding. Week after week, his clinical instructor gave him clinical assignments that involved caring for newborns who were in the neonatal intensive care unit because they were born opioid-addicted and were going through withdrawal. After more than a month of this, he said to his instructor that he would like to have a broader range of clinical experiences than he had been having. His clinical instructor replied that she could not place him with "normal families" and, according to him, berated him for asking. It would be inappropriate for him to care for "normal families," for in these families the mother was breastfeeding. She would not want a man, who knew nothing about breastfeeding, helping her; nor would her husband. My friend explained that his wife had breastfed their three children, an experience his fellow students did not have. Not only did his clinical instructor deny him the clinical experience he had asked for, she told him that he should never question a superior's decision like that again; he needed to take the assignments he was given. She placed him in the neonatal intensive care unit for the remainder of his clinical experience.

Women have the choice not to have a male obstetrician. When they give birth at a teaching hospital, they have the choice not to have male residents and interns see them. They should also be given the choice not to have a male nurse. However, to assume mothers (and fathers) would not want a male nurse denies them their right of choice. In this case, it also denied the male nursing student the chance to learn about all aspects of maternal–newborn nursing care.

Incivility, in word or deed, communicates disrespect for people because of difference—different genders, different races and ethnicities, different cultures and creeds, or different levels of experience. Sexism, racism, and other forms of discrimination and intolerance are not morally defensible and, hence, always result in incivility. We should not permit them in the civil community of nurses, and at times, we do have to take unpopular stances by calling them out.

Belief in human equality is at the root of civil behavior. Even when the working relationship is vertical, people higher up the vertical organizational chart show their moral belief in the equality of humanity by treating employees with civility and vice versa. Health care is not a democracy. Different providers have different scopes of practice and, thus, different responsibilities. Although we have our own licenses and practice autonomously within the scope of our licensure, we are fundamentally part of the broader scientific and health care communities. The kind of nursing community we create reflects on us in the broader communities of which we are a part. It is striking that we can be rated by the public as among the most honest and ethical of the professions, yet the extent of incivility among nurses is so great. At what point will this incivility bleed into our interactions with the other communities of which we are a part? At what point will other scientists and health care professionals and, most important, patients begin to witness our unequal treatment of each other?

Uncivil behavior lies in a person's perception of inequality. This perception may be the fear of having less power, or it may be the fear of ceding the power one has to another. Uncivil behavior is an attempt to gain (or keep) a power advantage; that is, one treats another uncivilly to make (or to keep) the relationship unequal—in favor of the one committing the incivilities. This, however, is a cynical view of life.

Cynicism is the belief that people are motivated solely by self-interest. We treat others uncivilly to get a leg up in our relationships with them—to overpower them—in an attempt to ensure our dominance. However, the contemporary psychologist Dacher Keltner has argued convincingly that humans have evolved not to be cynics but rather to live in communities in which we value resolution of conflicts, sympathy, and concern for others' welfare. Although hierarchical societal structures are part of human life, Keltner claims that, evolutionarily, survival favors the kindest. People rise to positions of importance when they "advance the interests of other group members." Rather than the cynical belief that I will only get ahead if I put down my colleague, "power," Keltner says, "goes to those who are socially engaged."

Uncivil behavior may originate from the perception that we lack, or may lose, status. The profession of nursing has a history of working within the hierarchies of health care that have treated the profession unequally. This history is the history of the typically male-dominated disciplines of medicine dominating the typically female-dominated discipline of nursing. Given this history, it is no wonder we nurses try to hold on to the power we have. Yet in turning our attempts onto ourselves, we enact among ourselves the very inequalities that have been enacted upon us. According to Keltner, studies have shown that "bullies, who resort to aggression, throwing their weight around, and raw forms of intimidation and dominance, in point of fact, are outcasts and low in the social hierarchy." This is the invidious nature of incivility: in our attempts to gain power for ourselves through uncivil behaviors, we disempower ourselves.

The power of the profession of nursing is based on its deep commitment to the equality of all people in the conditions necessary for a healthy life. Based on that commitment, it is our duty to show respect for all people. It is in our commitment to equality and our duty to respectful behaviors that we find the space to build the civil community of nursing. We journey with people at the most vulnerable times of their lives—through joyous and tragic births, through childhood diseases and development into adulthood, through chronic illnesses, and through dying. We care for people in these times. We care for them as people based on the respect that they are due as our equals in the human community. It is this same respect we owe each other as nurses.

The force of the profession of nursing to change the world for the better is great. In the United States, nursing is the largest profession among the health care professions, and among all the occupations in the United States, it is second in the number of people employed in it. We are many, and we touch many, many more lives.

To bring about the good society among the many lives we touch, we first must bring it about among ourselves. Our work to bring about the good society for all starts with bringing about the good society among the community of nurses, a community in which we treat all nurses with respect. Moreover, we continue to empower ourselves among other health care professions when we build a civil community for ourselves.

The good society is a vision of how the world *ought* to be. For nurses, it is a vision of equality in the conditions necessary for life and for that which sustains life. This vision cannot abide the divisions that come from disrespect, divisions that perpetuate inequality. We need to hold for ourselves the same vision of the good society that we hold for the world. Yet within our own community, we create divisions with our uncivil treatment of each other. Our uncivil treatment excludes our fellow nurses from fully inhabiting the space of the good society, a space in which the belief in the equality of humanity is held dear and lived by.

However, we can create this space for the good society among all nurses through civility. Fundamentally, civility demonstrates to others, in word and deed, our moral commitments. In the workplace, we must communicate to each other, through our respectful behaviors, our commitment to the equality of all nurses—that is, to the humanity of all nurses. Through civility, we create the space for us to be one indivisible community of nurses. Creating the space for a civil community is a habit of a good nurse.

Chapter 11

Being Grateful

You have wonderful times nursing. You attend births. You watch children grow up and, over the years, help them prevent and overcome illnesses. You provide care to patients in the intensive care unit, patients you thought had the medical facts stacked against them; but they recover. You watch a patient with a spinal cord injury regain the ability to walk. You hold on to these moments, these "miracle" moments. They keep you going.

You also have difficult times. You break the bad news to the 36-year-old woman pregnant for the first time that, alas, the lump she just found in her breast is cancerous. You tell the otherwise fit 50-year-old man that he did have a heart attack on the treadmill at the gym; it was not just acid reflux. Your 78-year-old patient in the intensive care unit who you thought would pull through takes a turn for the worse; she dies. Her husband of sixty years comes into the room. You spend thirty minutes comforting him. You have no control over how slow a clinic moves, but a patient screams at you for having to sit in the waiting room for an hour. You have six very sick patients on this shift, not one who can toilet unaided; it is going to be a long shift. These moments exhaust you physically and drag you down emotionally. You go home weary—a profound weariness. In these moments, it is hard to be aware of the good you do.

But you do good. You are a nurse, and the work you do as a nurse is good work. When you sat with the man who had just lost his wife, whom he loved and upon whom he depended, you did good. Yes, of course, you had five other patients to attend to. Yes, one of them had sat on a bedpan for far too long and, now because of this, you fear plummeting patient satisfaction scores. Being aware of the moments in which you gave of yourself, moments such as with the grieving husband, brings the difficulties of your work into the company of the good. Being aware of the good that you do places you in the presence of that which is good in your life.

It can be hard to be aware of the good of your life as a nurse. You face so many difficulties. To be sure, the difficulties of our work need proper redress. At times, we do need to shout about these difficulties all the way up to the decision makers. We do need work environments that are safe for us and for our patients, and we need to be rewarded, valued, and recognized for our work. However, amid all the difficulties of the work of nursing, it is good—that is, it is ethically significant—that you use your life professionally to promote and restore the health of others, even as they are dying and grieving. Your life, and your work as a nurse, is good. If there is only one thought you remember after reading this book, I hope it is the thought that being alive is good and that which promotes or restores aliveness is good.

Just because something is good does not mean that we all ought to act in a way to bring it about all the time. Pleasure, we all agree, is good; but we cannot all live in such a way that we seek our own pleasure at all times. The trash, after all, has to be taken out, the dishes washed, and the baby's diaper changed. Likewise, even though life is good, it is not the case that, say, in all circumstances, we must do all we can to keep a terminally ill patient alive. Rather, we as nurses promote and restore the health of others—and we work for others to have a serene death—because their lives are good. Life is good, and we do good when we provide nursing care that promotes or restores the aliveness of others, even as they are dying.

How, when you are done reading this book, can you think about the goodness of life? How, with the busyness and the difficulties of nursing, can you notice aliveness?

The answer is to be grateful.

When you are grateful, you notice those moments when you— or anyone—act to promote or restore aliveness. You delivered the woman you were midwifing of a healthy baby, and you were grateful. You caught the patient's arrhythmia on the telemetry monitor in time to prevent her death, and you were grateful. You were the nurse for the grandmother dying of ovarian cancer who, before she died, was able to fulfill her dream of dancing at her granddaughter's wedding; and you were grateful. We do not always expect moments of aliveness. But when these moments occur, being grateful for them causes us to remember that life is good.

Being grateful focuses our vision on the aliveness of our patients and what we do to promote it. My patient sat in the examining room listing to his right side, the side of his body that was almost completely paralyzed. He could stand with a balancing aid, but he could not walk. Nor could he use his right arm; it dangled at his side. He drooled out of the right side of his mouth, which curved downward. I had just listened to his lungs. They sounded "junky," to use a nontechnical term we all know. Junk in the lungs is never good. I suspected the muscles that control swallowing were going; his lungs were probably sucking into them whatever was meant to go down his throat into his stomach. His sister had brought him into the clinic because he was running a low-grade fever. Pneumonia was my fear: Knowing that my patient, who was only 25 years old, was dying of an advanced-stage, high-grade brain tumor, I sat down after performing the physical exam and told him and his sister, who was his only caregiver and just 28 years old herself, that I thought the time had come for him to go to the inpatient hospice, our plan for when the end was nigh. He had already made it clear that he did not want to be treated for an infection, should he get one. He had made clear in his advance directives that he did not want antibiotics but that he did want to be kept comfortable. I thought he had only a few days left to live, and sure enough, he died just a few days later. But that day, the day I had sat down next to him and told him and his sister that it was his time to die, he, slumping in the chair next to me, put out his left hand, his only working hand, and said, "Thank you."

I could not figure out what my patient had to be grateful for. His all-too-young life was coming to a quick close, and the last few years of it had been full of misery. He had wanted to become a professional sportsman. He played golf, and the year before the brain tumor was diagnosed, when he was just 21 years old, he had earned his Professional Golf Association (PGA) tour card. But he never played in a PGA tournament. One day, after a long stint of playing golf, he had a one-car accident. Police thought he was drunk, but the breath analyzer showed him to be free of alcohol. They took him to the hospital, where a magnetic resonance image of the brain showed a tumor. He had probably had a seizure on the road. Within two years, he would be dead. What did he have to be grateful for that day, when he knew that life was just about over?

There was no good in his disease—or in his prognosis. Death is always difficult. We recover some losses, but death is irrevocable. It is the deepest and most final of all losses. And yet, when I told this young man that his death lurked around the corner, he responded with gratitude for the honesty and respect I had shown him. In that difficult moment, my patient's gratitude brought me into the presence of the goodness of the work I had done to promote the life that he had. My patient brought me into the goodness of the work of nursing and into the goodness of my being a nurse. When we are grateful, we see that there are good things in the world, even when inexplicably bad things happen to good people. We notice the good of what we do as nurses to promote the aliveness of our patients, even as they are dying.

Sometimes, however, things go wrong. We make mistakes. When bad things happen in our nursing practice, we can learn from them and become better at promoting or restoring the aliveness of our patients. Amelia, the oncology nurse who transposed the numbers in a patient's weight that was used to calculate the patient's chemo-therapy dose, was horrified at her mistake. In her case, the mistake would have meant the patient would have gotten too low a dose of the medication, and it would not have been effective. If her mistake had been in the other direction, she could have set off a chain of events that, if unchecked by other staff, could have killed the patient. This scenario is not fiction. In 1994, a calculation error by a young physician at one of the world's leading cancer centers caused two patients to receive four times the correct amount of a chemotherapy medication. One patient died. The other patient sustained irrevers-ible heart damage. Twenty-five cancer center staff members involved in these patients' care did not notice the error until weeks later. There is nothing to be grateful for in the gross error that was made. However, reform came from the cancer center's and the profession's response to this error. Standards for chemotherapy ordering, dis-pensing, and administering changed for prescribers, pharmacists, and nurses. Patients are now better protected from harm, and health care providers are now better safeguarded against human fallibility. The error that was made, and the awful circumstances that came from it, can never be seen as good. However, the response, in mini-mizing the risk of harm and promoting the aliveness of patients yet to come, was good. Being grateful notices the good that comes from getting it right after we have made a mistake. Getting it right is central to being a good nurse. Getting it right is not just getting it correct. Getting it right means that we do what we must in order to become a good nurse, a nurse who notices that (and how) her or his nursing care is focused on promoting or restoring patients' aliveness. Being grateful about the times we get patient care right is to care about becoming a good nurse.

When we are grateful, we put a marker on the path of everyday life to indicate that we noticed the goodness of life. We mark moments of aliveness—our own moments of aliveness and our patients' moments of aliveness. We mark the times that, through our nursing care, we have promoted or restored the aliveness of our patients. And we mark those instances in which we have learned from our mistakes to become more proficient. When we are grateful, we memorialize the moments in which we are aware of the goodness of life.

The importance of letting others know we are grateful is that it makes others grateful, too. Other nurses help us with our difficult nursing tasks, and we are grateful. They provide that check for us; they keep our practice safe, and we are grateful. Other nurses cover us for fifteen minutes while we take a bathroom break or nosh on the granola bar that has gotten crushed in our pockets over the last six hours of our shift because we have not had a chance to eat it. When we are grateful for others' kindnesses toward us, we notice what they have done to sustain our lives. Being grateful for what others have done for us entails saying "thank you." "Thank you," after all, is not an empty expression. Expressing gratitude, the social psychologist Robert Emmons says, "requires us to see how we have been supported and affirmed by other people." Expressing gratitude is the recognition that we cannot be who we are—or do what we do—without the help of others.

I am not advocating a gratitude intervention, such as keeping a gratitude journal, in order to make us feel better about ourselves. Indeed, a 2016 meta-analysis of gratitude intervention studies found that, although gratitude interventions outperformed control groups in improving psychological well-being, the effect size was small. The authors of the meta-analysis concluded "that gratitude interventions may operate through placebo effects." Placebo effects occur when the people experiencing the intervention expect it to improve their condition. One might argue that it really does not matter whether gratitude interventions improve our psychological well-being by themselves or through placebo effects, as long as our psychological well-being improves. And so be it. Yet this is not the reason I suggest we are grateful.

We are grateful because, when we are, we become better nurses—and better people. We notice moments of aliveness, and then we seek to promote and restore aliveness through our everyday acts of nursing care. Just as all of a sudden we notice that spring has come and the trees have budded, so, too, when we notice the goodness of life, we are grateful for the people and circumstances in our lives that help us improve; and when we are grateful, we become better nurses. It is not as if bad things do not happen to us; of course they do. This is part of what it means to live in an imperfect world. The bad things of our nursing lives need addressing—fixing, insofar as they can be fixed. But being grateful changes what we notice. We move our vision away from the bad and fix it on the good we do as nurses—we promote and restore aliveness, even for the dying. Being grateful puts us in the presence of all the good that nurses do. Indeed, being grateful puts us in the presence of life itself.

Chapter 12

Toward a Better World

Nursing and ethics, according to Annie Goodrich, share the same nature, for what it means to be a good nurse and what it means to be a good person are inherently the same. So much is nursing of the same essence as ethics, Goodrich says, "that it is consistent to assert that the terms good and ethical as applied to nursing are synonymous." This synonymy rests in nursing and ethics sharing the same objective. For Goodrich, "life's ethical objective . . . is to produce a better world." Nursing's objective is the same: a good nurse works toward a better world. Throughout her book *The Social and Ethical Significance of Nursing*, Goodrich describes this better world as a world of peace and a world of equal access to good food, safe drinking water, adequate shelter, quality education, upward mobility, and high-quality health care. This better world is nursing's ultimate aim.

The eighteenth-century philosopher David Hume argued that we need a common point of view when speaking about how to act or about what needs to be done in order to bring about a better world. It may seem that working toward a better world begins with rational argument that sets forth rules or ethical principles. Curiously, however, we find that rules or principles derived through reasoning do not produce a better world. Goodrich herself bemoans the desire to formulate rules of ethical conduct, and she encourages us to see the impossibility of the task. Likewise, Hume did not think that we could achieve a common point of view through reason alone. We can use reason, after all, to argue that people with whom we disagree about what constitutes a better world or how to bring it about are ignorant or inferior, or we may think their principles for a better world are perverse; we may impose our desires on them, as authoritarian rule does; or we may manipulate or deceive them into cooperating with us to bring about our notion of a better world. In such instances, we use our reasoning skills and our own sets of rules or principles to exclude other, differing views from our idea of a better world. There is no common point of view to be achieved through reasoning alone. Hence, reasoning, and the principles that are derived from reasoning, do not serve as the foundation of ethics. Rather, as Simon Blackburn puts it, common concerns form the foundation of ethics.

I have argued throughout this book that, in nursing, caring anchors nursing ethics. Caring, not reasoned principles, enables us to work toward a better world. Reasoned principles act as incentives. But, as Goodrich says, being a good nurse "requires no goad of duty"; being a good nurse requires "utmost care." Caring about—and for—others is the beginning of a better world.

People do have reasons for wanting a better world. People suffer from war and want peace for very sound reasons. People want water for drinking and bathing free from parasites that cause blindness and from chemicals and minerals that cause irreparable physical harm. Expectant parents want an end to the Zika virus so that they do not have to fear their children being born with microcephaly. Parents want to be able to provide good nutrition for their growing children and for their children to be able to achieve what they want in life. People living with human immunodeficiency virus (HIV) and acquired immunodeficiency syndrome (AIDS), and the countless others affected by HIV and AIDS, want the virus rendered impotent. But these reasons do not form the basis for our moral response to others' needs. It can seem like the most awful banality if we who live in safety, plenty, and health come along and reassure those who suffer from these ills that we share their point of view, that their reasons are our reasons. As Blackburn puts it, "'I share your pain' is the sentimental drivel of the talk show." We will not achieve a better world merely by agreeing with another person's reasons for wanting a better world.

However, we as nurses can take up the concerns of others and make them our own. We cannot fully understand the patient who experienced war and now suffers from post-traumatic stress disorder. We cannot fully understand the patient who has neurologic complications from drinking lead-tainted water or who has gone blind from bathing in water infected with schistosomiasis. Nor can we fully understand the pain of the parents whose child was born with Zika-related microcephaly or get into the mind and the body of the patient who suffers from cancer-related pain. We can, however, care about their concerns. That is, caring about their concerns can be motivation for our nursing practice. In this way, the maladies of our patients can become our maladies, not literally but in the sense that we act out of a concern to improve their situation—indeed, out of a feeling of caring about them. What motivates us is not a set of reasons or a rational process that leads us to inviolable principles. What motivates us is caring. Caring for and about other human beings, and that which sustains human life, is the deep root of nursing ethics from which grows our acts of nursing care.

Caring is a way of life. We cannot merely say that we care or read about caring in a textbook, nodding our heads in agreement: we must live and practice in such a way as to show we care. Through our nursing practice we show to our patients and their communities, to our colleagues in nursing and in other health care professions, and to our families and friends that we care. Perhaps most important, we must show it to each other, for it is from nurses who care that we learn how to care.

I have learned how to care for people in the most intimate of ways from other nurses. I learned how to change a bed, protect patients from falling, give a back rub, and a bed-bath. I also learned that sometimes, when nothing else would do, sitting in silence at the patient's side is an act of caring. Patient by patient, family by family, I learned how to care about a better world from nurses who cared about a better world. In the process, I also learned that caring about a better world is not the result of reasoning about ethical rules or principles. It is a way of living and practicing in an imperfect world.

Patients and families know firsthand the imperfections of the world. We all do, for we all know what it is like to be sick. And we all know that, when we are sick, we are soothed by someone who cares for us. I shall never forget being in the hospital when I was twelve years old. I had broken my arm. It needed to be repaired by a specialist orthopedic surgeon, which my small town did not have. My parents took me to the nearest university hospital, a three-hour drive away. After the operation on my arm, my parents had to return home, to my younger siblings and to work. I remained in the hospital for a week. During that week, nurses cared for me as though I were their own child. My concerns became their concerns. They made the world, though imperfect, a better place for me. The world of patients and families is better than it would otherwise be because we care.

The habits of a good nurse, when practiced, show to our patients and their communities that we care. Consider how our trustworthiness brings about a better world for patients and families. Trustworthiness makes relationships possible. The balance of the relationship between the health care system and patients and families hangs unequally in the health care system's favor. Patients and families have less control and power over their care than those who understand the workings of the system, and they may not feel justified in trusting that system. However, through our trustworthiness, we are a conduit for relationships between patients and families and other providers in the health care system and thereby help to rebalance this unequal relationship.

Because we have proven ourselves trustworthy time and time again, patients believe what we say. We teach them how to care for their bodies, salve their wounds, bring down their fevers, nurse their young, and attend their dying loved ones. We tell them what their medications are and how they work. They listen, and because we have proven trustworthy before, they believe us. Indeed, most knowledge depends on trust. They believe the health care–related knowledge we give them because they have learned that they can trust us. This believability is the basis for patients' abilities to make decisions about their health care. They need to know what the options are and what these options mean. People base the believability of this knowledge on our trustworthiness. Moreover, when they make decisions, they believe that we will carry them out.

Caring involves imagination of what a better world might look like. We imagine a future for our patients that they may not be able to see for themselves, and then we care for them in such a way as to achieve that future, a future of the best health, or the most peaceful death, possible. Likewise, we imagine a world in which there is equal access to quality health care, then we work to that end. We imagine a world free from the social conditions that lead to disease: poverty, unclean water, unsafe food, the lack of public health infrastructures, a planet that is warming at a rate such that vector-borne diseases threaten health in a new and alarming way. We imagine an

environment that sustains health. We imagine the conditions necessary for safe births and schoolchildren vaccinated against diseases
that maim and kill. We imagine a world without war. We imagine
this better world, and this imagination drives our nursing practice.
We imagine a better world and, through the practice of nursing care,
bring it about—here and there, person by person, life by life.

In order to bring about a better world, we need to cultivate in
ourselves the habit of seeing the beauty of life—the beauty of the
life of our patients, their communities, and the earth that sustains
all life. In our daily work, we see the effects of disease and disorder.
We also see the effects of destruction and the despair of inhumanity.
We feel the fear of economic uncertainty and the instability of geo-
politics. These are injuries to society. However, through the habit of
seeing the beauty of all life, we project justice into these injuries and
promote the preservation of life and that which sustains life. The
habit of seeing beauty and according beauty the justice it deserves
is also the way nursing practice aims to bring about a better world.

We all share in the human condition, in which we are vulnerable
to disease and disorder, to natural disasters and accidents, and to
the degradation of that which sustains life. As nurses, we see our
patients' vulnerability, but also we see them as seeking a lessening
of their vulnerability. When we care, we create the space for a better
world in their lives. The space of care is the space in which patients
and families find the succor they need to resist vulnerability, even
during the uncertainty of disease and disorder. We all feel this
uncertainty. I knew a person who exercised faithfully, ate a healthful
diet of locally sourced organic foods—a person who did everything
right—and still developed life-limiting cancer. I know that sudden
cardiac death struck down an elite runner who was fitter than most
of us ever hope to be. People, merely by accident of their birth and,
thus, where they have to live, die of Ebola, through no fault of their

own. As nurses, we bring into this uncertainty the constancy of care, care that creates a space for a better world, if only for this patient and this family today, right now. The habit of creating space is the habit of projecting a better world into uncertainty and vulnerability.

By practicing the habits of a good nurse, we are the presence of a better world for our patients and their communities. Individual moments of care—a moment when we can be trusted, when we imagine a healthful and peaceful future for others, when we see the beauty of aliveness and create an inhabitable space—join with other moments of care to produce something larger and different from the imperfect world patients and families experience. When we practice the habits of a good nurse, we produce in the here and now a world that is better than disease and disorder, a world in which vulnerability and uncertainty are lessened. When we cultivate in ourselves the habits of a good nurse, we bring that which is good to the clinic, the hospital, the home, the school, the hospice—to the Earth we live on. In a most profound way, nursing presence is the presence of a better world, a presence found in each and every act of nursing care. Nursing presence, in this sense, is *being* for patients and their communities what they need you to be in order to produce a better world.

Nursing presence is powerful on the individual level. Each of us has the chance to be the bearer of a better world for the patients and families for whom we care. But collectively nursing has the power to present the vision of a better world to society at large. Among the professions that require specialized education and certification necessary to be employed, nursing has the largest employment in the United States. Given the power of numbers, not just in the United States but around the world, the profession of nursing is a large and powerful presence. The community of nurses, as a singular community across the globe, has the power to bring about a better world. With this power comes duty, duty insofar as the ultimate aim of nursing cannot be achieved without caring for and about people in such a way that works toward a better world. Indeed, the ethical significance of nursing rests in the acts of individual nurses caring for individual people, acts that cumulatively produce a better world in the here and now and work toward a better world for generations to come.

All that I have written in this book is not nursing ethics. Nursing ethics is not written, nor is it spoken. Nursing ethics is practiced. I hope that, after reading this book, you now see that the ethics of nursing rests not in reasoned principles but in your caring about a better world for people and in your caring for them in such a way that brings it about. In this book, I have discussed five habits: trustworthiness, imagination, beauty, space, and presence. When you practice these habits, be assured that, as a good nurse, you are working toward a better world for the people for whom you care.

NOTES

Foreword

x: Patricia Benner, Molly Sutphen, Victoria Leonard, and Lisa Day, *Educating Nurses, A Call for Radical Transformation* (San Francisco, CA: Jossey-Bass; Palo Alto, CA: Carnegie Foundation for the Advancement of Teaching, 2009).

x: Tom L. Beauchamp and James F. Childress, *Principles of Biomedical Ethics*, 7th ed. (New York: Oxford University Press, 2012).

xi: Onora O'Neill, *A Question of Trust: The BBC Reith Lectures 2002* (Cambridge, UK: Cambridge University Press, 2002).

xi: Virginia Henderson, "The Nature of Nursing," *American Journal of Nursing* 64 (1964): 62–67.

Chapter 1 — The Moral Character of Nursing

3:   See Donna Diers's definition of nusing as "caring for the sick or the potentially sick and tending the care environment" in her book *Speaking of Nursing ...: Narratives of Practice, Research, Policy, and the Profession* (Sudbury, MA: Jones and Bartlett Publishers, 2004), x.

3:   Aristotle, "Eudemian Ethics," trans. J. Solomon, in J. Barnes, ed., *The Complete Works of Aristotle*, Vol. 2 (Princeton, NJ: Princeton University Press, 1984), 1922–1981; "Nicomachean Ethics," trans. W. D. Ross, in J. Barnes, ed., *The Complete Works of Aristotle*, Vol. 2 (Princeton, NJ: Princeton University Press, 1984), 1729–1867.

4: Frederick Buechner, *Wishful Thinking: A Seeker's ABC*, rev. and exp. ed. (San Francisco, CA: HarperSanFrancisco, 1993), 119.

4: For the notion of an internal principle in ethics, see Immanuel Kant's work on the sublime, particularly Patrick R. Frierson and Paul Guyer, eds., *Immanuel Kant: Observations on the Feeling of the Beautiful and Sublime and Other Writings*, Cambridge Texts in the History of Philosophy (Cambridge, UK: Cambridge University Press, 2011).

5: Annie Warburton Goodrich, *The Social and Ethical Significance of Nursing: A Series of Addresses* (New Haven, CT: Yale University School of Nursing, 1932, Reprinted, 1973): "a new social order," p. 14; "a better world," p. 6; "a world not striven by war," p. 239; "delimiting border of countries . . . a common humanity," p. 261; "a world of equality for women and children," 261, 262–273; "no patient has to stay longer than is . . . necessary," 153.

5: See Ann Gallagher, "Editorial," *Nursing Ethics* 19 (2012): 3–4.

6: Patricia Benner, "A Dialogue Between Virtue Ethics and Care Ethics," *Theoretical Medicine* 18 (1997): 47–61; 57.

6–7: Adam Nossiter and Ben C. Solomon. "If They Survive in Ebola Ward, They Work On," *New York Times*, August 24, 2014, A1.

8: Tom L. Beauchamp and James F. Childress, *The Principles of Bioethics* (Oxford, UK; New York, NY: Oxford University Press, 1977).

8: On the notion of "right" as a relative term, see Ludwig Wittgenstein, "A Lecture on Ethics," *Philosophical Review* 74 (1965): 3–12.

9: Beauchamp and Childress, *Principles of Bioethics*, 26.

9: On the adjectival form of ethos, see: S. Sekine, *A Comparative Study of the Origins of Ethical Thought: Hellenism and Hebraism*, trans. J. Wakabayashi (Oxford, UK: Rowman & Littlefield, 2005).

11: Derek Sellman, *What Makes a Good Nurse: Why the Virtues Are Important for Nurses* (London, UK: Jessica Kingsley, 2011).

Chapter 2—Trustworthiness

17: Gallup, "Honesty/Ethics in Professions," accessed January 17, 2016, http://www.gallup.com/poll/1654/honesty-ethics-professions.aspx.

17: Rebecca Riffkin, "Americans Rate Nurses as Highest on Honesty, Ethical Standards," Gallup, accessed January 17, 2016, http://www.gallup.com/poll/180260/americans-rate-nurses-highest-honesty-ethical-standards.aspx.

18: Onora O'Neill, *A Question of Trust: The BBC Reith Lectures 2002* (Cambridge, UK: Cambridge University Press, 2002). See also Onora O'Neill, "What We Don't Understand About Trust," filmed June 2013 at TEDx HousesOfParliament, TED video, 09:50, accessed June 1, 2016, http://www.ted.com/talks/onora_o_neill_what_we_don_t_understand_about_trust/transcript?language=en.

19:   Patricia Benner, *From Novice to Expert: Excellence and Power in Clinical Nursing Practice* (Menlo Park, CA: Addison-Wesley, 1984).

20:   Gallup, "Honesty/Ethics in Professions."

21:   See Mark Lazenby, Ruth McCorkle, and Daniel P. Sulmasy, eds. *Safe Passage: A Global Spiritual Sourcebook for Care at the End of Life* (New York, NY: Oxford University Press, 2014).

23:   O'Neill, *A Question of Trust.*

24:   "fairness, n.". OED Online. June 2016. Oxford University Press. http://www. oed.com/view/Entry/67729?redirectedFrom=fairness (accessed August 25, 2016).

25:   Paolo Coelho, *Brida*, trans. Margaret Jull Costa (New York, NY: HarperCollins, 2008), 56.

26:   Frederick Buechner, *Wishful Thinking: A Seeker's ABC*, rev. and exp. ed. (San Francisco, CA: HarperSanFrancisco, 1993).

26:   Helen Nicholson, *The Knights Hospitaller* (Rochester, NY: Boydell Press, 2001).

Chapter 3—Imagination

29:   Throughout this chapter I am deeply indebted to the work of the philosopher Cora Diamond. See, in particular, her "Ethics, Imagination and the Method of Wittgenstein's Tractatus." In R. Heinrich and H. Vetter, eds., *Bilder der Philosophie: Reflexionen uber das Bildliche und die phantasie* (Vienna, Austria: R. Oldenbourg Verlag, 1991), 55–90.

33:   Carol Gilligan, *In a Different Voice: Psychological Theory and Women's Development* (Cambridge, MA: Harvard University Press, 1982).

34:   Ashley Folgo, PMHNP, DNP (c), personal conversation, January 13, 2016.

34:   Margaret Farley, *Compassionate Respect: A Feminist Approach to Medical Ethics and Other Questions* (Mawah, NJ: Paulist Press, 2002), 37–38.

36:   David Bromwich, *Moral Imagination: Essays* (Princeton, NJ: Princeton University Press, 2014), 12 and 21. On the importance of resistance to morality, see Carol Gilligan, "Moral Injury and the Ethic of Care: Reframing the Conversation About Differences," *Journal of Social Philosophy* 45 (2014): 89–106.

Chapter 4—Beauty

42:   St. Augustine, *Da Musica*, trans. W. F. Jackson Knight, in ed. Albert Hofstadter and Richard Kuhns, *Philosophy of Art and Beauty* (Chicago: University of Chicago Press, 1976), 196. Also quoted in Elaine Scarry, *On Beauty and Being Just* (Princeton, NJ: Princeton University Press, 1999), 24.

43:   Scarry, *On Beauty*, 24.

43: Elaine Scarry, "Beauty and the Pact of Aliveness," in Bandy Lee, Nancy Olson, and Thomas P. Duffy, eds., *Making Sense: Beauty, Creativity, and Healing* (New York, NY: Peter Lang, 2014), 27. This notion that injury, not ugliness, is the opposite of beauty is throughout Elaine Scarry's *The Body in Pain: The Making and Unmaking of the World* (New York, NY: Oxford University Press, 1985); see especially Chapter 2: "The Structure of War: The Juxtaposition of Injured Bodies and Unanchored Issues." See Margaret Farley, *Compassionate Respect: A Feminist Approach to Medical Ethics and Other Questions* (Mawah, NJ: Paulist Press, 2002), 71, for a discussion on injustice and suffering.

44: Annie Warburton Goodrich, *The Social and Ethical Significance of Nursing: A Series of Addresses* (New Haven, CT: Yale University School of Nursing, 1932, Reprinted, 1973), 26.

47: Simon Curtis, dir., *The Woman in Gold*, Film, Origin Pictures/BBC Films, 2015. See also Anne Marie O'Connor, *The Lady in Gold: The Extraordinary Tale of Gustav Klimt's Masterpiece, Portrait of Adele Bloch-Bauer* (New York, NY: Alfred A. Knopf, 2012).

48: Immanuel Kant, *Critique of Practical Reason*, trans. Mary J. Gregor (Cambridge, UK: Cambridge University Press, 1999), 133.

50: Goodrich, *Social and Ethical Significance*, 26.

51: Virginia Henderson, "The Nature of Nursing," *American Journal of Nursing* 64 (1964): 64.

53: Iris Murdoch, *The Sovereignty of the Good over Other Concepts: The Leslie Stephen Lecture* (Cambridge, UK: Cambridge University Press, 1967), 2. See Scarry, *On Beauty*, 112ff. See also Scarry's use of Murdoch in "Beauty and the Pact of Aliveness," 29.

Chapter 5—Space

55: I am indebted to the work of Judith Butler for this entire thought of space—or inhabitable space—as a habit. See Judith Butler, *Notes Toward a Performative Theory of Assembly* (Cambridge, MA: Harvard University Press, 2015).

57–58: On the notion of compassion as a driving emotion, see Martha Nussbaum's classic article, "Compassion: The Basic Social Emotion," *Social Philosophy and Policy* 13 (1996): 27–58.

59–61: I am thankful to Ronica Mukerjee, APRN, DNP (c), for a version of this clinical case.

62: Carol Gilligan, "Moral Injury and the Ethic of Care: Reframing the Conversation About Differences," *Journal of Social Philosophy* 45 (2014): 89–106.

Chapter 6—Presence

67: Margaret Farley, *Compassionate Respect: A Feminist Approach to Medical Ethics and Other Questions* (Mawah, NJ: Paulist Press, 2002), 40.
68: Farley, *Compassionate Respect*, 37.
69: See, for instance: Deborah Finfgeld-Connett, "Meta-Synthesis of Presence in Nursing," *Journal of Advanced Nursing* 55 (2006): 708–714.

Chapter 7—The Challenge of Unreasonable Demands

76: Simon Blackburn, *Being Good: A Short Introduction to Ethics* (New York, NY: Oxford University Press, 2001), 50.
78: The work of Linda Aiken has proven the points in this paragraph. In particular, see J. Silber et al., "Comparison of the Value of Nursing Work Environments in Hospitals Across Different Levels of Patient Risk," *Journal of the American Medical Association Surgery* 151 (2016): 527–536; and: M. McHugh et al., "Better Nurse Staffing and Nurse Work Environments Associated with Increased Survival on In-Hospital Cardiac Arrest Patients," *Medical Care* 54 (2016): 74–80.
79: See, for instance, Henry L. Roediger and Brigid Finn, "Getting It Wrong: Surprising Tips on How to Learn," *Scientific American*, October 20, 2009.
79: For an example of this, see Jacob Brix, "Fail Forward: Mitigating Failure in Energy Research and Innovation," *Energy Research and Social Science* 7 (2015): 66–77.
80: Torsten Wilholt, "Group Emotion and Group Understanding," in Michael S. Brady and Miranda Fricker, eds., *The Epistemic Life of Groups: Essays in the Epistemology of Collectives*, (New York, NY: Oxford University Press, 2016), 220.
82: Wilholt, "Group Emotion."
82: On the notion of health for all people, see the World Health Assemby's Resolution 34.38, 1981, as cited in Health as a Potential Contribution to Peace: Realities from the field: what has WHO learned in the 1990s." Available at: http://www.who.int/hac/techguidance/hbp/HBP_WHO_learned_1990s.pdf

Chapter 8—The Threat of Becoming Automatons

85: I have discussed this notion of nurses as automatons previously in my article "On the Humanities of Nursing," *Nursing Outlook* 61 (2013): e9–e14.
88: Alexandra Robbins, "The Problem with Satisfied Patients," *The Atlantic*, April 17, 2015, http://www.theatlantic.com/health/archive/2015/04/the-problem-with-satisfied-patients/390684/.
88: See also Alexandra Robbins, *The Nurses* (New York, NY: Workman Publishing, 2015).

Chapter 9—Being Good to Ourselves

103: Patrick R. Frierson and Paul Guyer, eds., *Immanuel Kant: Observations on the Feeling of the Beautiful and Sublime and Other Writings*, Cambridge Texts in the History of Philosophy (Cambridge, UK: Cambridge University Press, 2011).

Chapter 10—Creating a Civil Community

105: Marie A. Castronovo, Amy Pullizzi, and ShaKhira Evans, "Nurse Bullying: A Review and a Proposed Solution," *Nursing Outlook* 64 (2015): 208–214.

105: Christine Porath and Christine Pearson, "The Price of Incivility," *Harvard Business Review* 91 (2013): 114–121.

106: "civility, n.". OED Online. June 2016. Oxford University Press. http://www.oed.com/view/Entry/33581?redirectedFrom=civility (accessed August 25, 2016).

106: Cheshire Calhoun, "The Virtue of Civility," *Philosophy & Public Affairs* 29 (2005): 251–279; 259. Also see John Locke, *Some Thoughts Concerning Education*, §143, in Charles W. Elliott, ed., *The Harvard Classics*, 1st ed., Vol. 37 (New York, NY: Collier, 1937), 240.

108: John Rawls, *Theory of Justice* (Cambridge, MA: Harvard University Press, 1999), 179.

108: Rawls, *Theory of Justice*, 337–338.

111: Dacher Keltner, *Born to Be Good: The Science of a Meaningful Life* (New York, NY: W. W. Norton, 2009), 63–64.

112: Keltner, *Born to Be Good*, 64.

112: US Department of Labor, Bureau of Labor Statistics, "Occupational Employment Statistics: May 2015 Occupational Profiles," http://www.bls.gov/oes/current/oes_stru.htm.

Chapter 11—Being Grateful

120: Robert Emmons, "How Gratitude Can Help You Through Hard Times," Greater Good Science Center, May 13, 2013, http://greatergood.berkeley.edu/article/item/how_gratitude_can_help_you_through_hard_times. See also Robert A. Emmons and Robin Stern, "Gratitude as a Psychotherapeutic Intervention," *Journal of Clinical Psychology* 69 (2013): 846–855.

121: Donald E. Davis, Elise Choe, and Joel Meyers, "Thankful for the Little Things: A Meta-Analysis of Gratitude Interventions," *Journal of Counseling Psychology* 63 (2016): 20–31.

Chapter 12—Toward a Better World

123: Annie Warburton Goodrich, *The Social and Ethical Significance of Nursing: A Series of Addresses* (New Haven, CT: Yale University School of Nursing, 1932, Reprinted, 1973), 5.

123: David Hume, *Enquiries Concerning the Human Understanding and the Principles of Morals*, 3rd ed., edited by L. A. Selby-Bigge, revised by P. H. Nidditch (Oxford, UK: Oxford University Press, 1975).

124: Simon Blackburn, *Being Good: A Short Introduction to Ethics* (New York, NY: Oxford University Press, 2001), 129–133.

125: Goodrich, *Social and Ethical Significance*, 5.

125: Blackburn, *Being Good*, 132.

129: US Department of Labor, Bureau of Labor Statistics, "Occupational Employment Statistics: May 2015 Occupational Profiles," http://www.bls.gov/oes/current/oes_stru.htm.

130: See Ludwig Wittgenstein, "A Lecture on Ethics," *Philosophical Review* 74 (1965): 3–12.

BIBLIOGRAPHY

Augustine. "Da Musica." Translated by W. F. Jackson. In *Philosophy of Art and Beauty*, edited by Albert Hofstadter and Richard Kuhns. Chicago, IL: University of Chicago Press, 1976.

Aristotle. "Eudemian Ethics." Translated by J. Solomon. In *The Collected Works of Aristotle*, vol. 2, edited by Jonathan Barnes. Princeton, NJ: Princeton University Press, 1984.

Aristotle. "Nichomachean Ethics." Translated by W. D. Ross. In *The Collected Works of Aristotle*, vol. 2, edited by Jonathan Barnes. Princeton, NJ: Princeton University Press, 1984.

Beauchamp, Tom, and James Childress. *The Principles of Bioethics*. New York, NY: Oxford University Press, 1977.

Benner, Patricia. "A Dialogue Between Virtue Ethics and Care Ethics." *Theoretical Medicine* 18 (1997): 47–61.

Benner, Patricia. *From Novice to Expert: Excellence and Power in Clinical Nursing Practice*. Menlo Park, CA: Addison-Wesley, 1984.

Blackburn, Simon. *Being Good: A Short Introduction to Ethics*. New York, NY: Oxford University Press, 2001.

Brix, Jacob. "Fail Forward: Mitigating Failure in Energy Research and Innovation." *Energy Research and Social Science* 7 (2015): 66–77.

Bromwich, David. *Moral Imagination: Essays*. Princeton, NJ: Princeton University Press, 2014.

Buechner, Frederick. *Wishful Thinking: A Seeker's ABC*. Revised and expanded edition. San Francisco, CA: HarperSanFrancisco, 1993.

Butler, Judith. *Notes Toward a Performative Theory of Assembly*. Cambridge, MA: Harvard University Press, 2015.

Calhoun, Cheshire. "The Virtue of Civility." *Philosophy & Public Affairs* 29 (2005): 251–279.

Castronovo, Marie, Amy Pullizzi, and ShaKhira Evans. "Nurse Bullying: A Review and a Proposed Solution." *Nursing Outlook* 64 (2015): 208–214.

Coelho, Paolo. *Brida.* Translated by Margaret Jull Costa. New York, NY: HarperCollins, 2008.

Curtis, Simon, dir. *The Woman in Gold.* Film. Origin/BBC Pictures, 2015.

Davis, Donald, Elise Choe, and Joel Meyers. "Thankful for the Little Things: A Meta-Analysis of Gratitude Interventions." *Journal of Counseling Psychology* 63 (2016): 846–855.

Diamond, Cora. "Ethics, Imagination, and the Method of Wittgenstein's *Tractatus.*" In *Bilder der Philosophie: Reflexionen uber das Bildliche und die Phantasie,* edited by R. Heinrich and H Vetter. Vienna, Austria: R. Oldenbourg Verlag, 1991, 55–90.

Diers, Donna. *Speaking of Nursing . . .: Narratives of Practice, Research, Policy, and the Profession.* Sudbury, MA: Jones and Bartlett, 2004.

Emmons, Robert. "How Gratitude Can Help You Through Hard Times." Greater Good Science Center, May 13, 2013. Accessed January 17, 2016. http://greatergood.berkeley.edu/article/item/how_gratitude_can_help_you_through_hard_times.

Emmons, Robert, and Robin Stern. "Gratitude as a Psychotherapeutic Intervention." *Journal of Clinical Psychology* 69 (2013): 846–855.

Farley, Margaret. *Compassionate Respect: A Feminist Approach to Medical Ethics and Other Questions.* Mahwah, NJ: Paulist Press, 2002.

Finfgeld-Connett, Deborah. "Meta-Synthesis of Presence in Nursing." *Journal of Advanced Nursing* 55 (2006): 708–714.

Hume, David. *Enquiries Concerning the Human Understanding and the Principles of Morals,* 3rd ed. Edited by L. A. Selby-Bigge. Revised by P. H. Nidditch. Oxford, UK: Oxford University Press, 1975.

Gallagher, Anne. "Editorial." *Nursing Ethics* 19 (2012): 3–4.

Gallup. "Honesty/Ethics in Professions." Accessed January 17, 2016. http://www.gallup.com/poll/1654/honesty-ethics-professions.aspx.

Gilligan, Carol. *In a Different Voice: Psychological Theory and Women's Development.* Cambridge, MA: Harvard University Press, 1982.

Gilligan, Carol. "Moral Inquiry and the Ethic of Care: Reframing the Conversation About Differences." *Journal of Social Philosophy* 45 (2014): 89–106.

Goodrich, Annie. *The Social and Ethical Significance of Nursing.* New Haven, CT: Yale University School of Nursing, 1932. Reprinted 1973.

Henderson, Virginia. "The Nature of Nursing." *American Journal of Nursing* 64 (1964): 62–68.

Kant, Immanuel. *Critique of Pure Reason.* Translated by Mary J. Gregor. Cambridge, UK: Cambridge University Press, 1999.

Kant, Immanuel. *Observations on the Feeling of the Beautiful and the Sublime and Other Writings*. Edited and translated by Patrick Frierson and Paul Guyer. Cambridge, UK: Cambridge University Press, 2011.

Keltner, Dacher. *Born to be Good: The Science of a Meaningful Life*. New York, NY: W. W. Norton, 2009.

Lazenby, Mark. "On the Humanities of Nursing." *Nursing Outlook* 61 (2013): e9–e14.

Lazenby, Mark, Ruth McCorkle, and Daniel P. Sulmasy, eds. *Safe Passage: A Global Spiritual Sourcebook for Care at the End of Life*. New York, NY: Oxford University Press, 2014.

Locke, John. *Some Thoughts Concerning Education*. The Harvard Classics, 1st ed., vol. 37. Edited by Charles W. Elliott. New York, NY: Collier, 1937.

McHugh, Matthew, Monica Rochman, Douglas Sloane, Robert Berg, Mary Mancini, Vinay Nadkarni, Raina Merchant, and Linda Aiken; American Heart Association's Get with the Guidelines-Resuscitation Investigators. "Better Nurse Staffing and Nurse Work Environments Associated with Increased Survival on In-Hospital Cardiac Arrest Patients." *Medical Care* 54 (2016): 74–80.

Murdoch, Iris. *The Sovereignty of the Good over Other Concepts: The Leslie Stephen Lecture*. Cambridge, UK: Cambridge University Press, 1967.

Nicholson, Helen. *The Knights Hospitaller*. Rochester, NY: Boydell Press, 2001.

Nossiter, Adam, and Ben C. Solomon. "If They Survive in Ebola Ward, They Work On," *New York Times*, August 24, 2014, A1.

Nussbaum, Martha. "Compassion: The Basic Social Emotion." *Social Philosophy and Policy* 13 (1996): 27–58.

O'Connor, Anne Marie. *The Lady in Gold: The Extraordinary Tale of Gustav Klimt's Masterpiece, Portrait of Adele Bloch-Bauer*. New York, NY: Alfred A. Knopf, 2012.

O'Neill, Onora. *A Question of Trust: The BBC Reith Lectures 2002*. Cambridge, UK: Cambridge University Press, 2002.

O'Neill, Onora. "What We Don't Understand About Trust," filmed June 2013 at TEDxHousesOfParliament, TED video, 09:50. Accessed July 5, 2016. http://www.ted.com/talks/onora_o_neill_what_we_don_t_understand_about_trust/transcript?language=en.

Oxford English Dictionary, 3rd ed. Oxford, UK: Oxford University Press, 2010.

Porath, Christine, and Christine Pearson. "The Price of Incivility." *Harvard Business Review* 91 (2013): 114–121. Accessed July 5, 2016. https://hbr.org/2013/01/the-price-of-incivility/.

Rawls, John. *A Theory of Justice*. Cambridge, MA: Harvard University Press, 1999.

Riffkin, Rebecca. "Americans Rate Nurses as Highest on Honesty, Ethical Standards." Gallup, December 18, 2014. Accessed January 17, 2016. http://www.gallup.com/poll/180260/americans-rate-nurses-highest-honesty-ethical-standards.aspx.

Robbins, Alexandra. *The Nurses*. New York, NY: Workman Publishing, 2015.

Robbins, Alexandra. "The Problem with Satisfied Patients." *The Atlantic*, April 17, 2015. Accessed July 5, 2016. http://www.theatlantic.com/health/archive/2015/04/the-problem-with-satisfied-patients/390684/.

Roediger, Henry, and Brigid Finn. "Getting It Wrong: Surprising Tips on How to Learn," *Scientific American*, October 20, 2009. Accessed July 5, 2016. http://www.scientificamerican.com/article/getting-it-wrong/.

Scarry, Elaine. "Beauty and the Pact of Aliveness." In *Making Sense: Beauty, Creativity, and Healing*, edited by Bandy Lee, Nancy Olson, and Thomas P. Duffy, eds. New York, NY: Peter Lang, 2014, 27–43.

Scarry, Elaine. *On Beauty and Being Just*. Princeton, NJ: Princeton University Press, 1999.

Scarry, Elaine. *The Body in Pain: The Making and Unmaking of the World*. New York, NY: Oxford University Press, 1985.

Sekine, Seizo. *A Comparative Study of the Origins of Ethical Thought: Hellenism and Hebraism*. Translated by Judy Wakabayashi. Oxford, UK: Rowman & Littlefield, 2005.

Sellman, Derek. *What Makes a Good Nurse: Why the Virtues Are Important for Nurses*. London, UK: Jessica Kingsley, 2011.

Silber, Jeffrey, Paul Rosenbaum, Matthew McHugh, Justin Ludwig, Herbert Smith, Bijan Niknam, Orit Even-Soshan, Lee Fleisher, Rachel Relz, and Linda Aiken. "Comparison of the Value of Nursing Work Environments in Hospitals Across Different Levels of Patient Risk." *Journal of the American Medical Association Surgery* 151 (2016): 527–536.

US Department of Labor, Bureau of Labor Statistics. "Occupational Employment Statistics: May 2015 Occupational Profiles." Accessed July 5, 2016. http://www.bls.gov/oes/current/oes_stru.htm.

Wilholt, Torsten. "Group Emotion and Group Understanding." In *The Epistemic Life of Groups: Essays in the Epistemology of Collectives*, edited by Michael S. Brady and Miranda Fricker. New York, NY: Oxford University Press, 2016.

Wittgenstein, Ludwig. "A Lecture on Ethics." *Philosophical Review* 74 (1965): 3–12.

World Health Organization. World Health Assembly Resolution 34.38, 1981. Accessed July 5, 2016. http://www.who.int/hac/techguidance/hbp/HBP_WHO_learned_1990s.pdf

DISCUSSION QUESTIONS AND EXERCISES

Chapter 1—The Moral Character of Nursing

1. Why did you choose nursing as a career? Did you feel called to nursing? If not, has a sense of calling grown as you practiced nursing?
2. Were the nurses who threatened the life of the head nurse in the Ebola ward in West Africa good nurses? Would you have volunteered to care for Ebola patients? Why or why not? Would you be a good nurse if you refused to care for Ebola patients? Why or why not?
3. How would you describe the moral character of nursing?
4. Think about a nurse you would like to emulate. What is it about that nurse that makes you want to practice like her or him?

Chapter 2—Trustworthiness

1. How can a novice nurse, though not competent, demonstrate her or his trustworthiness to patients?
2. What is the ethical impact on patients when a nurse says she or he will do something but does not do it?
3. What ought the profession's response be to nurses who are dishonest about aspects of patient care? What if the nurse intentionally gave a patient the wrong medication? What if the nurse withheld information?

4. What ought the profession's response be to nurses who commit unintentional medical errors that could have—or did—cause harm to patients?

Chapter 3—Imagination

1. Describe situations in which you have experienced the feeling of caring for a patient you had no connection with, other than being the patient's nurse.
2. Can you imagine a situation in which you would not provide care for a patient? How would refusal of care be ethical in this situation?
3. Discuss ways in which your imagination of yourself as a nurse helps you to become the nurse you wish to be. How does your imagination change the way you practice?

Chapter 4—Beauty

1. Describe an instance in which you, at first, could not think of the patient or the patient's loved ones as beautiful. Describe the ugliness of the situation. How could you have used nursing imagination to find beauty in the patient or the patient's loved ones?
2. How can we use the fine arts (the visual arts, music, theater, dance, creative writing, and so on) in our workplaces with patients and their communities to increase appreciation for aliveness?
3. The *Ars moriendi*, two related texts from the fifteenth century, talk about the art of dying well—even the beauty in dying, death, and grief. Today, we do not often talk about the art of dying well. However, can you describe a death you attended that was artful—beautiful? How was aliveness promoted in this instance?

Chapter 5—Space

1. Have you ever unwittingly—or at least without malice aforethought—made the place of care an uninhabitable space for one of your patients—or for your patient's loved ones? What can you do, after you have realized your mistake, to make the place of care a space the patient—or the patient's loved ones—can inhabit?

2. In our ever-smaller world, we find ourselves caring for patients and families from other cultures and nations. Sometimes we cannot even speak the same language and have to rely on translators, most often who are not there in person, to communicate with our patients and their families. How can you, amid the barriers of differing cultures and languages, still create a space in the place of care for them?

3. Suppose you hold beliefs that put you at odds with what a patient wants from your nursing care. Describe ways you and your nursing colleagues can create the space your patient needs without violating your own space to be true to yourself.

Chapter 6—Presence

1. Describe a moment in which you felt fully present to your patient. What were you aware of in this moment? How can you practice in such a way that you can replicate this moment with other patients?

2. When you are present to a patient, you respect that patient's ability to make decisions. What is involved in respecting a patient's decision, even though you may disagree with it?

3. What is the nature of your relationship with patients? How does this relationship change, if it all, with patients you feel an affinity for? What about with patients you struggle to like?

Chapter 7—The Challenge of Unreasonable Demands

1. Have you ever made a mistake like the one Amelia made? What did you do when you realized your mistake? Did you tell your nurse manager? Did you tell your patient? If so, did you feel more trustworthy after admitting your mistake?

2. If you made a mistake and never told anyone, do you feel as if you are still keeping a secret you are not willing to admit to others? How could admitting your mistake, even long after the fact, help you to feel more (indeed, help you to be) trustworthy?

3. How does admitting your mistakes help the community of nurses to be more trustworthy for each other? No one wants to make errors. No one wants one's nursing care to lead to harm. So within the bounds of our desire not to make mistakes, what is the nursing community's responsibility to individual nurses?

Chapter 8—The Threat of Becoming Automatons

1. Describe the ways in which technology helps you to feel as if your practice is safer, and describe the ways in which you feel technology impedes your ability to deliver personalized care to patients. How does the concept of nursing imagination help you to bridge these two, such that technology helps, not impedes, your ability to care?
2. Do you feel constrained by the power of the patient survey? Are you afraid that doing good for your patient may at times result in a survey response by a patient that casts your care in a negative light? How can you use nursing imagination to anticipate these moments and address them with your patient?

Chapter 9—Being Good to Ourselves

1. When have you not been good to yourself as a nurse? Describe the incident(s) (or reasons) that caused you not to be good to yourself. Now tell at least one of these incidents (or reasons) to a trusted friend or colleague. Tell the story in such a way that you end the story with justice, even with the justice of your surviving to tell the story.
2. Have you ever been cared for by a nurse in such a way that made you feel, well, cared for? Do you think the nurse who made you feel cared for saw the beauty of her or his care as a nurse? How can we as a nursing community help each other to see our own beauty?
3. Describe the ways in which you promote (or wish to promote) your own health—physical, emotional, and spiritual health. Does promoting your own health help you to see yourself as being fully alive?

Chapter 10—Creating a Civil Community

1. Describe the ways in which another nurse's uncivil behavior toward you has caused you to feel unwelcomed in the workplace. On what moral grounds do you have the right to respond to this nurse?
2. Have you found yourself being uncivil toward another nurse? According to the statistics, nearly all of us has. How can you correct yourself when you find yourself being uncivil or when another nurse has told you that you have been uncivil? What are the moral implications of doing nothing to correct your own behavior?
3. What are patient- and family-centered reasons that nurses should demonstrate civility to other nurses?

Chapter 11—Being Grateful

1. Keep a gratitude journal for at least three shifts in which you provide nursing care. At the end of each shift, write down at least ten things you were grateful for in your work as a nurse. By the end of the exercise, were you more aware of the good that you did? Were you more aware of the need to show your gratitude to others?
2. Describe an instance in which a patient or another nurse expressed gratitude to you. How did this make you feel? In what ways did it make you more aware of the good that you do as a nurse?

Chapter 12—Toward a Better World

1. When you hear of great tragedies around the globe, such as a devastating Ebola outbreak or hundreds of migrants leaving the coasts of North Africa on dinghies and drowning in the Mediterranean Sea, what is your inward response as a nurse? What should the profession of nursing's response be to these global tragedies?
2. How do you, in your work as a nurse, demonstrate to your patients and their communities that you care about making the world a better place?

INDEX